GOOD ENERGY AND VITALITY

TRANSFORMING YOUR HEALTH WITH EVERYDAY HABITS

DR. JESSICA REEVES

TABLE OF CONTENT

CHAPTER 15

THE JOURNEY AHEAD

- Setting Long-term Goals
- Staying Motivated and Focused
- Embracing the Continuous Journey of Health and Vitality

Chapter 1

WHAT YOU NEED TO KNOW ABOUT ENERGY AND VITALITY

What Does It Mean to Have Energy and Vitality?

It is energy that serves as the basis for life.

Energy is the fundamental energy that gives all living creatures their drive and enables them to carry out the myriad of activities that are necessary for their continued existence. In human health, energy may be regarded as the capacity to undertake physical, mental, and emotional tasks. To a large extent, it is obtained from the foods that we consume, and it is quantified in terms of calories. The body's capacity to convert these calories into usable energy depends on various factors, including metabolism, the effectiveness of cellular activities, and the balance of nutrients consumed.

Vitality: Going Beyond the Level of Physical Health

The term **"vitality"** refers to a condition of robust physical and mental well-being characterized by excitement, passion for life, and resilience. Vitality includes a wider spectrum than simply energy. Although energy is a component of vitality, genuine vitality also requires a harmonic balance of physical health, mental clarity, emotional stability, and a feeling of purpose. However, vitality is not the same thing as energy. It represents an individual's whole life energy and their potential to flourish, not merely survive.

The Interconnection of Energy and Vitality

The relationship between energy and vitality is inextricably intertwined, with one affecting the other. Sufficient energy levels enable the body to conduct everyday activities successfully, while vitality ensures these actions are undertaken with excitement and vigor. On the other hand, a lack of energy can result in exhaustion, which in turn lowers an individual's vitality and general quality of life satisfaction. Achieving and sustaining maximum energy and vitality needs a comprehensive strategy that addresses multiple elements of health and lifestyle.

The Importance of Balanced Energy in Daily Life

Balanced energy levels are vital for sustaining productivity, minimizing burnout, and boosting general well-being. Fluctuations in energy levels can lead to tiredness, trouble focusing, and diminished motivation. By recognizing and regulating elements that impact energy—such as diet, physical exercise, sleep, and stress—individuals may attain a more stable and prolonged energy supply, supporting improved performance in all aspects of life.

Factors Influencing Energy and Vitality

1. **Nutrition:** The quality and content of the food greatly affect energy levels and vitality. Consuming a balanced diet rich in whole foods, including fruits, vegetables, lean meats, and healthy fats, offers the required elements to promote energy generation and general health.

2. **Physical Activity:** Regular exercise raises energy levels by improving cardiovascular health, boosting muscular function, and encouraging efficient metabolic processes. Physical activity also adds to brain clarity and emotional well-being.

3. **Sleep:** Adequate and restful sleep is crucial for replenishing energy and preserving vigor. Poor sleep quality or inadequate sleep can contribute to persistent exhaustion, reduced cognitive performance, and diminished emotional resilience.

4. **Stress Management:** Chronic stress depletes energy reserves and badly influences vitality. Effective stress management practices, such as mindfulness, meditation, and relaxation exercises, assist in maintaining a healthy balance of energy.

5. **Mental and Emotional Health:** A positive mental state and emotional balance are key for preserving energy and vitality. Engaging in activities that foster mental clarity, emotional stability, and a feeling of purpose increases overall well-being.

How Vitality Impacts Overall Well-being

Vitality is a fundamental measure of overall well-being, indicating an individual's capacity to experience life to the fullest. High vitality levels are related to greater physical health, better stress management, higher cognitive function, and a more optimistic view of life. Individuals with high vitality are more robust, able to cope with adversities successfully and experience higher joy and contentment.

In contrast, low vitality can lead to several negative effects, including persistent weariness, greater susceptibility to sickness, emotional instability, and a lower quality of life. By prioritizing habits that boost energy and vitality, individuals may greatly improve their overall health and well-being, leading to a more vibrant and satisfying existence.

The Importance of Balanced Energy in Daily Life

Balanced energy is crucial for sustaining general well-being and ensuring that individuals can execute everyday chores quickly and successfully. It is not just about having bursts of high energy but about retaining a steady level of energy throughout the day. This balance fosters physical, mental, and emotional health, enabling individuals to lead productive, satisfying lives.

1. Enhancing Productivity and Performance

Balanced energy levels are vital for effective performance in both personal and professional situations. When energy is well-regulated, individuals can concentrate better, think more clearly, and finish things more effectively. This leads to increased productivity, whether at a job, school, or home.

Points:

- Improved attention and concentration.
- Increased efficiency in work completion.
- Enhanced problem-solving and decision-making ability.

2. Preventing Burnout and Fatigue

Maintaining balanced energy helps prevent the physical and mental tiredness associated with burnout. It lets individuals prolong their activities without feeling unduly weary or agitated, encouraging long-term health and well-being.

Points:

- Reduces the risk of persistent tiredness.

- Helps control stress levels.
- Promotes sustainable work-life balance.

3. Supporting Physical Health

Balanced energy levels help to enhance physical health by ensuring the body has sufficient fuel to conduct various duties. This encompasses everything from regular physical activity to crucial functions like digestion and immunological response.

Points:

- Enhances physical endurance and strength.
- Supports metabolic health and weight management.
- Boosts immune function and overall physical resiliency.

4. Improving Mental and Emotional Well-being

Energy balance strongly influences mental and emotional well-being. Consistent energy levels help regulate mood, reduce anxiety, and increase general mental clarity. This creates an optimistic mindset and emotional resiliency.

Points:

- Stabilizes mood and decreases mood swings.
- Decreases anxiety and depression symptoms.
- Enhances cognitive function and mental clarity.

5. Promoting Healthy Sleep Patterns

Balanced energy levels are intimately connected to sleep quality. Proper energy management throughout the day encourages better sleep at night, which in turn helps control energy levels for the following day. This cyclical link underlines the significance of a comprehensive approach to energy balance.

Points:

- Supports normal sleep habits.
- Improves sleep quality and duration.
- Reduces sleep disruptions and insomnia.

6. Fostering Social and Interpersonal Relationships

When individuals have balanced energy levels, they are more likely to engage favorably in social relationships. They may participate actively in social events, develop stronger connections, and enjoy higher levels of social happiness.

Points:

- Enhances social involvement and participation.
- Improves communication and relationship-building abilities.
- Increases contentment and fulfillment in social relationships.

Practical Strategies for Maintaining Balanced Energy

1. Nutrition:

- Eat a well-rounded diet that includes a variety of nutrients.
- Avoid excessive sugar and processed carbs.
- Ensure every meal includes protein, healthy fats, and fiber.

2. Physical Activity:

- Engage in frequent, moderate exercise.
- Incorporate both aerobic and strength-training routines.
- Avoid lengthy periods of idleness.

3. Sleep:

- Aim for 7-9 hours of quality sleep each night.
- Maintain a regular sleep routine.
- Create a comfortable sleep environment.

4. Stress Management:

- Practice mindfulness and relaxation practices.
- Manage time effectively to decrease stress.
- Seek help when required.

5. Hydration:

- Drink lots of water throughout the day.
- Limit coffee and alcohol consumption.

- Monitor hydration levels, especially during strenuous exertion.

6. Mental and Emotional Health:

- Engage in activities that improve mental well-being.
- Foster healthy relationships and social ties.
- Seek professional treatment for mental health difficulties when necessary.

Balanced energy is vital for having a healthy, productive, and satisfying life. By employing measures to maintain constant energy levels, individuals can boost their physical health, mental clarity, emotional stability, and general quality of life. Prioritizing balanced energy is a fundamental step in achieving long-term well-being and vitality.

How Vitality Impacts Overall Well-being

Vitality, frequently characterized as the ability for a bright and active existence, extends beyond basic physical health. It involves mental, emotional, and social well-being, leading to a holistic feeling of living completely and efficiently. Understanding how vitality influences overall well-being is critical for anybody wanting to create a balanced and meaningful life.

1. Enhancing Physical Health

Vitality substantially impacts physical health by encouraging an active lifestyle and fostering healthy body functioning. Individuals with high vitality are more likely to engage in regular physical exercise, maintain a nutritious diet, and adopt practices that support their physical well-being.

Points:

- Increased Physical Activity: Higher energy levels permit more consistent exercise, which improves cardiovascular health, strengthens muscles, and boosts flexibility.
- Improved Immune Function: Vitality promotes a healthy immune system, lowering the frequency and severity of infections.
- Better Weight Management: Vital persons frequently have a regulated metabolism, assisting in maintaining a healthy weight.

2. Boosting Mental Clarity and Cognitive Function

Mental vigor is defined by acute cognitive ability, fast reasoning, and an active mind. It helps to superior problem-solving abilities, creativity, and the capacity to learn and adapt.

- Enhanced Cognitive Performance: Regular mental stimulation and a healthy lifestyle promote greater brain function and memory retention.
- Reduced Risk of Cognitive Decline: Active mental engagement can lessen the risk of neurodegenerative disorders like Alzheimer's.
- Improved Focus and Concentration: Vitality helps sustain focus and clarity, making daily chores easier and more effective.

3. Promoting Emotional Stability

Emotional vitality refers to a condition of emotional balance and resilience, where individuals can effectively handle stress, cope with problems, and retain a positive attitude.

Points:

- Better Stress Management: High-vitality folks have more powerful coping mechanisms and recover from stress more rapidly.
- Positive Mood and Outlook: Vitality creates a positive attitude, minimizing the occurrence of anxiety and sadness.
- Greater Emotional Resilience: Resilient individuals can bounce back from losses and maintain emotional stability.

4. Strengthening Social Connections

Vitality increases social well-being by promoting healthier connections and enhancing social involvement. Individuals with high vitality tend to be more gregarious, empathic, and attached to their communities.

Points:

- Increased Social Interaction: High energy and excitement stimulate more social activities and better personal connections.
- Improved Communication Skills: Vitality fosters greater listening, empathy, and understanding, boosting interpersonal connections.
- Community Engagement: Vital persons are more likely to join in community activities, adding to a sense of belonging and purpose.

5. Enhancing Longevity and Quality of Life

Overall vitality is intimately connected to lifespan and a higher quality of life. Individuals who maintain high levels of vitality tend to live longer, healthier, and more meaningful lives.

Points:

- Extended Lifespan: Vital persons frequently have better lives, which leads to a longer life expectancy.
- Improved Quality of Life: With greater physical health, mental clarity, emotional stability, and strong social ties, individuals have a higher quality of life.
- Greater existence Satisfaction: Vitality leads to a more full existence, with individuals feeling more productive and fulfilled.

Strategies to Enhance Vitality

1. Balanced Nutrition:

- Consume a diet abundant in whole foods, such as fruits, vegetables, lean proteins, and healthy fats.
- Avoid processed meals and excessive sugar.

2. Regular Physical Activity:

- Engage in a mix of aerobic, strength, and flexibility activities.
- Stay active throughout the day with hobbies like walking, gardening, or yoga.

3. Quality Sleep:

- Ensure 7-9 hours of peaceful sleep every night.
- Establish a consistent sleep schedule and establish a calming sleep environment.

4. Stress Management:

- Practice mindfulness, meditation, and relaxation techniques.
- Balance work and relaxation to avoid burnout.

5. Social Engagement:

- Cultivate meaningful connections and participate in social activities.
- Volunteer and connect with community groups.

6. Mental Stimulation:

- Keep the mind engaged with puzzles, reading, and acquiring new skills.
- Stay interested and open to new experiences.

7. Emotional Health:

- Practice appreciation and positive thinking.
- Seek professional help when required for emotional concerns.

Vitality is a cornerstone of total well-being, including physical health, mental clarity, emotional stability, and social relationships. By nourishing vitality via balanced living and proactive health initiatives, individuals may increase their quality of life, prolong their lifetime, and feel more joy. Embracing behaviors that promote vitality is key to establishing a lively and active existence, eventually contributing to comprehensive well-being.

Chapter 2

NUTRITION FOR SUSTAINED ENERGY

The Role of a Balanced Diet

A balanced diet is crucial for keeping energy levels throughout the day and maintaining overall health. It offers the vital nutrients required for the body's numerous processes, including energy generation, cellular repair, and proper functioning of organs and systems. Understanding the significance of a balanced diet in energy management is critical for obtaining and sustaining vitality and well-being.

1. Understanding Macronutrients

Carbohydrates: The Primary Energy Source

Carbohydrates are the body's principal source of energy. They are broken down into glucose, which feeds body processes and physical activities. Complex carbs, such as whole grains, legumes, and vegetables, deliver a continuous release of glucose into the circulation, helping to maintain constant energy levels.

Points:

- Complex Carbohydrates: These give sustained energy and minimize spikes and dips in blood sugar levels.
- Fiber: Found in whole grains, fruits, and vegetables, fiber aids with digestion and helps regulate energy release.

Proteins: Essential for Repair and Growth

Proteins are vital for healing tissues, developing muscles, and sustaining immunological function. While not a primary energy source, proteins play a role in preserving energy by supporting muscle mass and metabolic activities.

Points:

- High-Quality Proteins: Include lean meats, poultry, fish, eggs, dairy products, and plant-based sources such as beans and lentils.
- Amino Acids: Essential for tissue healing and immunological functions.

Fats: Concentrated Energy Providers

Fats are a concentrated source of energy and are vital for absorbing fat-soluble vitamins (A, D, E, and K). Healthy fats, such as those from avocados, nuts, seeds, and olive oil, enable continuous energy release and general wellness.

Points:

- Unsaturated Fats: Opt for sources like avocados, nuts, seeds, and olive oil.
- Omega-3 Fatty Acids: Found in fish and flaxseeds, they enhance heart health and cognitive function.

2. Importance of Micronutrients

Vitamins and Minerals: Crucial for Energy Generation

Micronutrients, including vitamins and minerals, serve critical roles in energy generation and general health. For example, B vitamins are needed for turning carbs into useful energy, while iron is essential for oxygen delivery in the blood.

Points:

- B-Vitamins: Found in whole grains, meats, and leafy greens, they are crucial for energy metabolism.
- Iron: Present in red meat, beans, and fortified cereals, iron is vital for energy and minimizing weariness.

Antioxidants: Protecting Cells from Damage

Antioxidants help protect cells from damage caused by free radicals, which can impair energy levels and general health. Foods high in antioxidants include fruits, vegetables, nuts, and seeds.

Points:

- Vitamin C and E: Found in fruits like oranges and greens like spinach, they help battle oxidative stress.
- Phytonutrients: Present in colored fruits and vegetables, these substances enhance general health and vitality.

3. Hydration: A Key Component of Energy Management

The Role of Water in Energy Levels

Adequate hydration is vital for sustaining energy levels and general health. Water is involved in several body activities, including digestion, nutrition absorption, and temperature regulation.

Points:

- Daily Water Intake: Aim for at least 8 glasses of water each day, adjusted for activity level and climate.
- Hydration and Performance: Dehydration can lead to weariness, poor focus, and diminished physical performance.

Electrolytes: Maintaining Fluid Balance

Electrolytes, such as sodium, potassium, and magnesium, assist control fluid balance and muscle performance. Consuming meals high in these minerals aids hydration and sustained energy.

Points:

- Sources of Electrolytes: Include bananas, oranges, spinach, and yogurt.

4. Timing and Frequency of Meals

Regular Meals and Snacks: Maintaining Energy Levels

Eating regular meals and snacks helps maintain steady blood sugar levels and prevents energy drops. Balancing meals with a combination of macronutrients and micronutrients offers sustained energy throughout the day.

Points:

- Meal Frequency: Aim for three balanced meals and one to two snacks daily.
- Balanced Snacks: Include a balance of protein, healthy fats, and complex carbs.

Avoiding Extreme Diets: The Importance of Moderation

Extreme dieting or missing meals can lead to swings in energy levels and metabolic abnormalities. It's crucial to develop a sensible and sustainable approach to eating that promotes long-term energy and health.

Points:

- Avoid Fad Diets: Focus on a well-rounded, nutrient-dense diet.
- Listen to Your Body: Eat when hungry and stop when full.

5. Personalizing Your Diet for Optimal Energy

Individual Nutritional Needs: Tailoring to Specific Requirements

Each person's nutritional demands may differ based on characteristics such as age, gender, activity level, and health problems. Personalizing your diet to fit these demands can assist boost energy levels and general health.

Points:

- Consultation with a Professional: Consider working with a licensed dietitian or nutritionist to build a tailored dietary plan.

- Adjusting for Health Conditions: Modify your diet based on specific health issues or dietary limitations.

A healthy diet plays a critical role in preserving energy levels and supporting overall health. By ingesting a range of macronutrients and micronutrients, staying hydrated, and scheduling meals efficiently, individuals may sustain constant energy throughout the day. Personalized food choices, guided by individual requirements and tastes, further increase energy levels and contribute to a lively and healthy life.

Superfoods for Energy and Vitality

Superfoods are nutrient-dense foods recognized for their extraordinary health benefits and potential to improve energy levels and vitality. These foods are rich in important vitamins, minerals, antioxidants, and other bioactive components that enhance general well-being. Incorporating superfoods into your diet will help maintain prolonged energy, increase immunological function, and promote overall vitality.

1. Leafy Greens: Powerhouses of Nutrition

Spinach

Spinach is filled with iron, magnesium, and vitamins A, C, and K. Iron is vital for energy generation and battling weariness, while magnesium helps muscular function and relaxation.

Benefits:

- Energy Production: High iron concentration assists in oxygen transport and energy metabolism.
- Antioxidant Defense: Abundant in antioxidants that safeguard cells against oxidative stress.

Kale

Kale is a great source of vitamins A, C, and K, as well as fiber and calcium. Its strong antioxidant concentration aids cleansing and general wellness.

Benefits:

- Vitality Boost: Nutrient-dense, supplying critical vitamins and minerals.
- Digestive Health: High fiber content improves digestion and intestinal health.

2. Berries: Nutrient-Rich Fruits

Blueberries

Blueberries are recognized for their strong antioxidant content, particularly anthocyanins, which help protect cells from harm and enhance cognitive function.

Benefits:

- Cognitive Support: Antioxidants boost memory and brain function.
- Anti-inflammatory Properties: Reduces inflammation and enhances overall health.

Goji Berries

Goji berries are rich in vitamins A and C, antioxidants, and amino acids. They are recognized for their immune-boosting effects and capacity to raise energy levels.

Benefits:

- Immune Support: High in antioxidants and vitamins that enhance the immune system.
- Energy Enhancement: Provides prolonged energy and combats weariness.

3. Nuts and Seeds: Nutrient-Dense Snacks

Almonds

Almonds are an excellent source of protein, healthy fats, and vitamin E. They assist sustain energy levels and improve heart health.

Benefits:

- Energy Sustainment: Provides protein and healthy fats for sustained energy.
- Heart Health: Contains heart-healthy lipids and antioxidants.

Chia Seeds

Chia seeds are abundant in omega-3 fatty acids, fiber, and protein. They help balance blood sugar levels and give long-lasting energy.

Benefits:

- Blood Sugar Regulation: High fiber content helps balance blood sugar levels.
- Omega-3 Fatty Acids: Supports brain function and decreases inflammation.

4. Whole Grains: Sustained Energy Providers

Quinoa

Quinoa is a complete protein source containing all nine necessary amino acids. It is also abundant in fiber, B vitamins, and minerals including magnesium and iron.

Benefits:

- Complete Protein: Provides all needed amino acids for energy and muscle repair.
- Nutrient-Rich: High in fiber and minerals that boost overall vigor.

Oats

Oats are a wonderful source of complex carbs and soluble fiber. They assist in maintaining consistent energy levels and improve digestive health.

Benefits:

- Steady Energy: Complex carbs give sustained energy throughout the day.
- Digestive Health: Soluble fiber aids healthy digestion.

5. Healthy Fats: Essential for Energy and Vitality

Avocado

Avocados are rich in monounsaturated fats, which improve heart health and provide a consistent supply of energy. They also include vitamins and minerals that boost general well-being.

Benefits:

- Heart Health: Monounsaturated fats enhance cardiovascular health.
- Nutrient-Dense: Contains vitamins, minerals, and antioxidants.

Coconut Oil

Coconut oil includes medium-chain triglycerides (MCTs) that are easily turned into energy. It also has antibacterial qualities that enhance general health.

Benefits:

- Quick Energy Source: MCTs give immediate energy and assist metabolism.
- Antimicrobial Properties: Supports immunological health and general vigor.

6. Herbs and Spices: Enhancing Energy and Health

Turmeric

Turmeric includes curcumin, a strong anti-inflammatory and antioxidant substance. It helps joint health, decreases inflammation, and enhances overall vigor.

Benefits:

- Anti-inflammatory: Reduces inflammation and improves joint health.
- Antioxidant Protection: Protects cells from oxidative damage.

Ginger

Ginger contains natural anti-inflammatory and digestive effects. It assists with digestion, improves the immune system, and helps maintain energy levels.

Benefits:

- Digestive Health: Supports healthy digestion and minimizes nausea.
- Immune Support: Boosts the immune system and decreases inflammation.

Incorporating Superfoods into Your Diet

Meal Planning Tips:

- Smoothies: Add berries, spinach, and chia seeds to smoothies for a nutritious boost.
- Salads: Top salads with almonds, avocado, and a variety of leafy greens.

- Snacks: Enjoy nuts and seeds as snacks or in homemade energy bars.
- Main Dishes: Use quinoa as a basis for salads or bowls and include turmeric and ginger in curries and soups.

Balancing Superfoods:

While superfoods offer several advantages, it is crucial to have a balanced diet that includes a range of foods. Combining superfoods with other nutrient-dense meals gives a holistic approach to health and vigor.

Superfoods are essential supplements to a balanced diet, delivering a multitude of nutrients that promote prolonged energy, vitality, and general well-being. By including a varied selection of superfoods in your regular meals, you may increase your health, improve energy levels, and promote long-term vitality. Embrace these nutrient-dense meals to feed your body and mind, and enjoy the advantages of a bright and active existence.

Meal Planning and Smart Eating Habits

Effective meal planning and sensible eating habits are vital for maintaining optimal health, preserving energy levels, and attaining long-term wellness objectives. By following these principles, individuals may make educated food choices, limit portion sizes, and guarantee a balanced intake of key nutrients. This systematic approach not only helps physical health but also enhances general well-being.

1. Benefits of Meal Planning

1.1. Improved Nutritional Intake

Meal planning helps consumers pick a range of nutrient-dense meals, guaranteeing a balanced diet of vitamins, minerals, proteins, fats, and carbs. This assists in reaching daily dietary needs and improves overall wellness.

Benefits:

- Nutrient Balance: Incorporates a varied range of foods to cover all key nutrients.
- Prevention of Deficiencies: Reduces the danger of nutritional deficiencies by maintaining a well-rounded diet.

1.2. Time and Cost Efficiency

Planning meals helps expedite grocery shopping and saves food wastage. By developing a grocery list based on scheduled meals, folks may purchase exactly what is required, saving time and money.

Benefits:

- Reduced Food Waste: Minimizes extra purchases and leftovers.
- Cost Savings: Helps budget better and minimizes impulsive buying.

1.3. Better Portion Control

Meal planning helps portion management by helping individuals to prepare balanced meals and prevent overeating. It also aids in regulating calorie intake and keeping a healthy weight.

Benefits:

- Controlled Portions: Ensures optimum serving amounts for balanced nutrition.
- Weight Management: Supports healthy weight by avoiding overeating.

2. Components of a Balanced Meal

2.1. Macronutrients

A balanced meal should have a healthy mix of macronutrients: carbs, proteins, and fats. Each plays a key part in energy generation, muscle repair, and general body processes.

Points:

- Carbohydrates: Opt for complex carbohydrates like whole grains, veggies, and legumes for sustained energy.
- Proteins: Include lean sources such as poultry, fish, legumes, and tofu for muscle regeneration and satiety.
- Fats: Choose healthy fats from avocados, nuts, seeds, and olive oil for energy and cell function.

2.2. Micronutrients

Incorporate a variety of fruits and vegetables to give critical vitamins and minerals. These micronutrients assist immunological function, bone health, and general vitality.

Points:

- Vitamins and Minerals: Focus on a colorful range of food to guarantee a broad spectrum of nutrients.
- Antioxidants: Include berries, leafy greens, and cruciferous vegetables to counteract oxidative stress.

2.3. Hydration

Adequate hydration is necessary for healthy health and energy levels. Incorporate water-rich meals and keep a constant water consumption throughout the day.

Points:

- Hydrating Foods: Include fruits and vegetables with high water content, such as cucumbers and melons.
- Daily Water Intake: Aim for at least 8 glasses of water every day, modifying based on activity levels and environment.

3. Smart Eating Habits

3.1. Eating Mindfully

Practice mindful eating by paying attention to hunger signs, appreciating each mouthful, and avoiding distractions during meals. This strategy assists in identifying actual hunger and preventing overeating.

Points:

- Mindful Eating: Focus on the sensory experience of eating and listen to your body's hunger and fullness signals.
- Avoid Distractions: Eat without multitasking to better assess satisfaction and enjoyment.

3.2. Balanced Snacking

Incorporate nutritious snacks between meals to maintain energy levels and prevent excessive hunger. Choose snacks that mix protein, fiber, and healthy fats.

Points:

- Healthy Snack alternatives: Consider alternatives like Greek yogurt with fruit, almonds, and seeds, or vegetable sticks with hummus.
- Portion Control: Avoid big snacks and opt for reasonable servings to maintain balanced energy.

3.3. Preparing Meals in Advance

Meal planning may save time and ensure you have nutritional alternatives readily available. Prepare and portion meals for the week, then store them in airtight containers for convenience.

Points:

- Batch Cooking: Prepare big quantities of essentials like grains, meats, and veggies for quick assembly over the week.
- Storage: Use proper containers to keep food fresh and conveniently accessible.

3.4. Adapting to Lifestyle and Preferences

Customize your meal plan to meet your lifestyle, dietary choices, and health objectives. Consider considerations including activity level, dietary limitations, and personal taste while preparing meals.

Points:

- Personalization: Tailor meal programs to meet individual requirements and tastes, assuring enjoyment and sustainability.
- Flexibility: Allow for tweaks and replacements based on availability and changing needs.

4. Overcoming Common Challenges

4.1. Managing Time Constraints

Busy schedules may make meal planning tough. Utilize time-saving tactics such as batch cooking, fast recipes, and utilizing kitchen appliances like slow cookers or pressure cookers.

Strategies:

- Batch Cooking: Prepare numerous meals at once to save time over the week.
- Quick Recipes: Opt for easy, healthful dishes that can be made in 30 minutes or less.

4.2. Navigating Social Situations

Social engagements and dining out might affect food planning. Plan by checking menus and choosing healthier choices, and don't hesitate to carry your snacks or meals if required.

Strategies:

- Menu Review: Check restaurant menus in advance and pick healthier alternatives.
- Social Flexibility: Be prepared to make modifications whether dining out or attending activities.

Effective meal planning and wise eating habits are crucial components of a healthy lifestyle, contributing to prolonged energy, adequate nutrition, and overall well-being. By concentrating on balanced meals, integrating nutrient-dense foods, and adopting mindful eating practices, individuals may achieve their health objectives and enjoy a bright, active existence. Embrace these ideas to establish a sustainable approach to eating that meets both your immediate and long-term health demands.

Chapter 3

THE POWER OF HYDRATION

Benefits of Staying Hydrated

Hydration is a cornerstone of health and well-being, impacting practically every area of human function. Water, representing roughly 60% of the human body, serves a fundamental function in maintaining physiological balance, supporting metabolic activities, and guaranteeing general vitality. Understanding the benefits of being hydrated can help individuals maximize their health and boost their everyday functioning.

1. Enhancing Physical Performance

1.1. Improved Exercise Efficiency

Proper hydration is necessary for healthy physical performance. Adequate fluid levels improve cardiovascular function, control body temperature, and sustain muscular function, which can boost endurance and strength during activity.

Benefits:

- Enhanced Endurance: Adequate hydration helps sustain energy levels and prevent the onset of exhaustion.

- Better muscular Function: Prevents muscular cramping and facilitates effective contraction and relaxation.

1.2. Faster Recovery

Hydration assists in the healing process following physical exertion. Water aids the replacement of fluids lost via perspiration, helps in the elimination of metabolic waste products, and minimizes the risk of dehydration-related ailments.

Benefits:

- Efficient Recovery: Accelerates the replenishment of lost fluids and aids muscle regeneration.
- Reduced Injury Risk: Helps avoid dehydration-related symptoms such as cramping and dizziness.

2. Supporting Cognitive Function

2.1. Enhanced Mental Clarity

Staying hydrated is vital for sustaining cognitive function. Dehydration can affect focus, memory, and general mental efficiency. Proper hydration improves brain function and keeps cognitive functions working properly.

Benefits:

- Improved Concentration: Supports attention and mental alertness.
- Better Memory: Enhances short-term memory and cognitive functioning.

2.2. Mood Regulation

Hydration influences mood and emotional well-being. Dehydration can contribute to irritation, anxiety, and mood swings, whereas regular fluid intake helps preserve emotional stability.

Benefits:

- Stable Mood: Reduces the likelihood of mood disruptions and promotes overall emotional equilibrium.
- Reduced Stress: Helps control stress levels and increases emotional resiliency.

3. Supporting Digestion and Nutrient Absorption

3.1. Efficient Digestion

Water is crucial for gut health. It assists in the digestion of meals, promotes nutrient absorption, and helps reduce constipation by softening feces.

Benefits:

- Digestive Efficiency: Facilitates the digestion and absorption of minerals.
- Constipation Prevention: Supports regular bowel motions and minimizes the risk of constipation.

3.2. Detoxification

Hydration contributes to the detoxification process by improving renal function and the removal of waste materials from the body. Adequate fluid consumption promotes the body's natural cleansing systems and helps maintain general health.

Benefits:

- Effective Detoxification: Enhances the elimination of toxins and waste products through urine.
- Healthy Kidney Function: Supports the kidneys in filtering and excreting waste.

4. Maintaining Healthy Skin

4.1. Skin Hydration and Elasticity

Proper hydration leads to healthy, vibrant skin. Water helps preserve skin hydration, suppleness, and overall look, decreasing the appearance of fine lines and dryness.

Benefits:

- Moisturized Skin: Keeps skin moisturized and supple.
- Improved Appearance: Reduces dryness and encourages a young complexion.

4.2. Preventing Skin Disorders

Adequate fluid consumption can help avoid skin disorders such as acne and eczema by maintaining skin hydrated and supporting overall skin health.

Benefits:

- Prevention of Skin Conditions: Reduces the incidence of skin disorders due to dryness and dehydration.
- Healthy Skin Function: Supports the skin's barrier function and resilience.

5. Regulating Body Temperature

5.1. Temperature Control

Water plays a significant function in controlling body temperature through the processes of sweating and evaporation. Proper hydration helps maintain a constant internal temperature, especially during strenuous exertion or hot weather.

Benefits:

- Effective Cooling: Supports the body's capacity to cool down via sweating.
- Temperature Regulation: Helps maintain a stable body temperature in different environmental situations.

5.2. Preventing Heat-Related Illnesses

Adequate hydration minimizes the incidence of heat-related disorders such as heat exhaustion and heat stroke by providing effective temperature control and fluid balance.

Benefits:

- Heat Illness Prevention: Minimizes the risk of heat-related diseases via proper hydration.
- Improved Thermoregulation: Enhances the body's capacity to regulate temperature swings.

6. How to Stay Hydrated

6.1. Daily Water Intake Recommendations

The standard recommended for daily water intake is roughly 8 glasses (2 liters) per day, while individual needs may vary based on factors such as age, activity level, and environment.

Recommendations:

- Individual Needs: Adjust water consumption depending on personal characteristics and lifestyle.
- Hydration Monitoring: Pay attention to thirst and urine color as signs of hydration status.

6.2. Hydrating Foods and Beverages

Incorporate water-rich meals such as fruits and vegetables into your diet. Additionally, herbal teas and infused waters can give diversity and boost hydration.

Recommendations:

- Water-Rich Foods: Include fruits like watermelon and cucumbers, and vegetables like lettuce and celery.
- Varied Beverages: Drink herbal teas and flavored waters to diversify fluid intake.

6.3. Managing Dehydration

Be careful of indicators of dehydration, such as dark urine, dry mouth, and weariness. Address dehydration quickly by increasing fluid intake and avoiding excessive coffee or alcohol.

Recommendations:

- Recognize Symptoms: Be mindful of dehydration signs and symptoms.
- Increase Fluid Intake: Drink water and hydrating fluids when suffering signs of dehydration.

Staying hydrated is vital for sustaining overall health and well-being. The benefits of optimum hydration extend to greater athletic performance, improved cognitive function, successful digestion, healthy skin, and efficient body-temperature management. By implementing techniques to maintain proper fluid intake and including water-rich foods in your diet, you may support your body's optimal functioning and live a bright, healthy life. Prioritize water as a crucial element of your daily health routine to enjoy the full spectrum of its advantages.

Hydration Strategies for Optimal Energy

Effective hydration is crucial to maintaining appropriate energy levels and general health. Proper fluid intake promotes several biological processes, including energy generation, mental clarity, and physical performance. Implementing strategic hydration strategies can boost vitality, avoid weariness, and improve everyday functioning. Here are some professional tips to help you keep appropriately hydrated for lasting energy.

1. Understand Your Hydration Needs

1.1. Daily Water Intake Recommendations

The usual recommended daily water intake is roughly 8 glasses (2 liters) per day. However, individual hydration needs might differ based on factors such as age, weight, exercise intensity, and environment.

Points:

- Individual Variability: Adjust fluid intake depending on personal circumstances and lifestyle.
- Hydration Goals: Aim to drink at least 2 liters of water every day, or more if needed based on activity levels and ambient circumstances.

1.2. Monitor Hydration Status

Pay attention to symptoms of hydration status, such as urine color and thirst. Clear or light-colored urine normally indicates appropriate hydration, but dark urine might be an indication of dehydration.

Points:

- Urine Color: Use urine color as a basic measure of hydration. Aim for pale yellow.

- Thirst Awareness**: Drink water regularly, even if you do not feel thirsty.

2. Incorporate Hydrating Foods

2.1. Water-Rich Fruits and Vegetables

Include fruits and vegetables with high water content in your diet to enhance hydration. Options such as watermelon, cucumbers, oranges, and strawberries boost fluid consumption and give additional nutrients.

Points:

- Fruits: Include water-rich fruits including watermelon, oranges, and apples.
- veggies: Add hydrating veggies such as cucumbers, celery, and lettuce.

2.2. Balanced Meals with Hydrating Components

Design meals that contain a combination of hydrating foods and beverages. Combining these with your regular meals will assist in maintaining constant water levels and improve overall energy.

Points:

- Salads and Soups: Incorporate salads and soups with high-water-content foods.

- Snack Options: Choose snacks like fruit salads and veggie sticks.

3. Strategic Beverage Consumption

3.1. Water as the Primary Hydrator

Water should be your major source of hydration. It is calorie-free and necessary for maintaining fluid balance and boosting energy levels.

Points:

- Regular Intake: Drink water consistently throughout the day, not only when thirsty.
- Hydration Habits: Carry a water bottle to remind yourself to drink regularly.

3.2. Hydration from Herbal Teas and Infused Waters

Herbal teas and infused waters may bring variation to your hydration regimen. These beverages provide an extra taste and can contribute to your daily fluid consumption.

Points:

- Herbal Teas: Opt for caffeine-free herbal teas, such as chamomile or peppermint.

- Infused Waters: Add fruits, herbs, or vegetables to water for a natural taste.

3.3. Be Cautious with Caffeine and Alcohol

While moderate caffeine use might aid in hydration, large quantities can have a diuretic impact. Similarly, drinking can cause dehydration. Balance these beverages with proper water consumption.

Points:

- Moderation: Consume caffeinated beverages and alcohol in moderation.
- Compensation: Drink more water to counterbalance the drying effects of coffee and alcohol.

4. Hydration during Physical Activity

4.1. Pre-Hydration

Drink water before commencing physical activities to ensure you begin exercising in a hydrated state. This helps prepare your body for the demands of exercise and decreases the danger of dehydration.

Points:

- Pre-Exercise Hydration: Consume 8-16 ounces of water around 1-2 hours before exercising.
- Hydration Goals: Adjust pre-exercise hydration based on the duration and intensity of the activity.

4.2. Hydration during Exercise

For exercises lasting longer than 60 minutes, try consuming electrolyte-enriched drinks to restore lost minerals and maintain hydration levels.

Points:

- Electrolyte Drinks: Use sports drinks or electrolyte solutions during lengthy exercises.
- Regular Sips: Drink water or electrolytes consistently while activity, generally every 15-20 minutes.

4.3. Post-Exercise Rehydration

Replenish fluids lost during exercise by drinking water and ingesting drinks with electrolytes. This helps restore fluid balance and aids recuperation.

Points:

- Post-Workout Hydration: Drink water and electrolyte drinks after exercise to rehydrate.
- Recovery meals: Include hydrated meals as part of your post-exercise meal.

5. Hydration for Special Conditions

5.1. Adapting to Climate

Adjust your hydration strategies based on environmental variables. In hot or humid situations, increase fluid intake to compensate for greater sweat loss.

Points:

- Hot Weather: Drink more water and consume hydrating meals at high temperatures.
- Cold Weather: Maintain hydrated in chilly climates, as dehydration can still develop in dry, cold air.

5.2. Hydration for Health Conditions

Certain health issues, such as diabetes or renal ailments, may necessitate particular hydration regimens. Consult with healthcare providers to adjust hydration methods to your requirements.

Points:

- Medical Advice: Seek counsel from healthcare specialists for hydration recommendations unique to your health circumstances.
- Customized Hydration: Adjust fluid consumption depending on physician advice and individual health needs.

Implementing good hydration methods is vital for maintaining healthy energy levels and general wellness. By recognizing your hydration needs, adding hydrating meals, eating suitable drinks, and adjusting to physical and environmental situations, you may boost your vitality and well-being. Prioritize continuous hydration as part of your daily routine to maintain prolonged energy, increase physical performance, and promote overall health.

Recognizing and Preventing Dehydration

Dehydration occurs when the body loses more fluids than it takes in, affecting normal physiological activities. It can range from moderate to severe and profoundly impair overall health and well-being. Recognizing the indications of dehydration and following preventative actions is vital for maintaining appropriate hydration and preventing potential health complications. This article contains vital information on identifying dehydration and techniques to prevent it.

1. Recognizing Dehydration

1.1. Common Symptoms of Dehydration

1.1.1. Thirst

A basic sign of dehydration is persistent thirst. The body indicates the need for fluid intake when hydration levels are low.

Symptoms:

- Increased Thirst: Feeling particularly thirsty or dry mouth.

1.1.2. Urine Changes

Changes in urine color and frequency are important symptoms of dehydration. Dark yellow or amber-colored urine frequently suggests insufficient fluid consumption, but lower urine flow may signal dehydration.

Symptoms:

- Dark Urine: Urine that is darker than light yellow.
- Reduced Frequency: Less frequent urinating than normal.

1.1.3. Dry Skin and Mucous Membranes

Dehydration may cause skin to become dry and lose its suppleness. Additionally, dry mucous membranes in the mouth and nose are prominent indications.

Symptoms:

- Dry Skin: Lack of moisture or suppleness in the skin.
- Dry Mouth: Sticky or dry feeling in the mouth and throat.

1.1.4. Fatigue and Dizziness

Insufficient fluid levels can contribute to symptoms of weariness, dizziness, and lightheadedness owing to lower blood volume and electrolyte imbalances.

Symptoms:

- Fatigue: Feeling especially weary or weak.
- Dizziness: Lightheadedness or feeling faint.

1.1.5. Headaches

Dehydration can contribute to headaches or migraines when the brain momentarily shrinks from fluid loss, leading to tension and pain.

Symptoms:

- Headaches: Persistent or recurring headaches.

1.1.6. Reduced Sweat Production

A considerable reduction in sweating can be a symptom of dehydration, especially in hot or physically taxing settings.

Symptoms:

- Less Sweat: Reduced perspiration during strenuous exercise or in heated surroundings.

1.2. Severe Dehydration Indicators

1.2.1. Confusion or Irritability

In severe situations, dehydration can impact cognitive function, leading to disorientation, irritability, or difficulty concentrating.

Symptoms:

- Confusion: Disorientation or trouble thinking clearly.
- Irritability: Increased moodiness or emotional instability.

1.2.2. Rapid Heartbeat and Breathing

Severe dehydration can induce an accelerated heart rate and fast breathing as the body tries to adjust for lower blood volume.

Symptoms:

- Rapid Heartbeat: Noticeably rapid or irregular heartbeat.
- Rapid Breathing: Increased pace of breathing.

1.2.3. Sunken Eyes and Dry Mouth

Sunken eyes and severely dry mouth are key indications of severe dehydration requiring quick attention.

Symptoms:

- Sunken Eyes: Deeply sunken eyes with a hollow look.
- Severe Dry Mouth: Intense dryness with trouble swallowing.

1.2.4. Low Blood Pressure

Severe dehydration can lead to a reduction in blood pressure, resulting in dizziness or fainting.

Symptoms:

- Low Blood Pressure: Feelings of dizziness or fainting upon standing.

2. Preventing Dehydration

2.1. Adequate Fluid Intake

2.1.1. Daily Water Consumption

Aim for roughly 8 glasses (2 liters) of water each day, adjusting for individual needs based on activity level, age, and ambient circumstances.

Recommendations:

- Regular Hydration: Drink water regularly throughout the day.
- Individual Needs: Adjust fluid consumption based on personal circumstances and exercise levels.

2.1.2. Include Hydrating Foods

Incorporate water-rich items such as fruits and vegetables into your diet to enhance hydration levels.

Recommendations:

- Water-Rich Foods: Consume fruits like watermelon and veggies like cucumbers.
- Balanced Meals: Include hydrated foods in meals and snacks.

2.2. Strategic Beverage Choices

2.2.1. Opt for Water

Water is the greatest alternative for maintaining hydrated without extra calories or sweets. Prioritize water as your major source of hydration intake.

Recommendations:

- Primary Fluid: Use water as the major source of hydration.
- Carry a Bottle: Keep a water bottle with you to encourage frequent drinking.

2.2.2. Limit Dehydrating Beverages

Limit the intake of caffeinated and alcoholic beverages, which can have diuretic effects and lead to dehydration.

Recommendations:

- Moderate Caffeine: Consume caffeinated beverages in moderation.
- Limit Alcohol: Drink alcohol safely and follow with appropriate water.

2.3. Hydration during Physical Activity

2.3.1. Pre-Exercise Hydration

Drink water before physical activity to achieve optimal hydration levels before exercise.

Recommendations:

- Pre-Workout: Consume 8-16 ounces of water 1-2 hours before exercising.

- Hydrate Early: Avoid commencing activity in a dehydrated state.

2.3.2. Hydrate during Exercise

For lengthy physical exercise, drink water often and consider electrolyte-enriched drinks to maintain hydration and electrolyte balance.

Recommendations:

- Regular Sips: Drink water every 15-20 minutes throughout continuous exertion.
- Electrolytes: Use sports drinks for activity lasting longer than an hour.

2.4. Adapting to Environmental Conditions

2.4.1. Hot and Humid Conditions

Increase fluid intake in hot or humid weather to compensate for excessive sweat loss and prevent dehydration.

Key Recommendations:

- Increased Intake: Drink additional water in hot or humid situations.
- Monitor Hydration: Adjust fluid intake based on temperature and activity level.

2.4.2. Cold Weather Considerations

Maintain hydrated in chilly weather, since dry air and reduced thirst can still contribute to dehydration.

Recommendations:

- Hydrate in Cold Weather: Continue to consume water despite reduced thirst in cold surroundings.
- Monitor Fluid Loss: Be cognizant of hydration demands even in frigid circumstances.

Recognizing and avoiding dehydration is crucial for preserving health and well-being. By knowing the indicators of dehydration and applying good hydration techniques, individuals may support their body's needs, increase energy levels, and prevent potential health complications. Prioritize regular fluid intake, add hydrating meals, and tailor hydration practices to activity levels and environmental circumstances to support adequate hydration and overall vigor.

Chapter 4

EXERCISE AND PHYSICAL ACTIVITY

Choosing the Right Exercise Routine

Selecting the correct workout program is vital for reaching optimal health, maintaining energy levels, and boosting general well-being. A successful exercise plan should correspond with individual objectives, interests, and physical capabilities while fostering long-term sustainability. This chapter covers crucial variables to consider when establishing an exercise regimen and gives suggestions on developing a balanced and pleasant fitness plan.

1. Assess Your Fitness Goals

1.1. Define Your Objectives

Understanding your fitness objectives is the first step in picking a suitable workout regimen. Goals might vary significantly, from weight loss to muscle building to improving cardiovascular health or strengthening flexibility.

Goals:

- Weight Loss: Focus on aerobic workouts and strength training to burn calories and develop lean muscle.

- Muscular Gain: Emphasize resistance training with increasing stress to enhance muscular growth.
- Cardiovascular Health: Incorporate aerobic workouts such as jogging, cycling, or swimming.
- Flexibility and Balance: Include stretching exercises or disciplines like yoga or Pilates.

1.2. Consider Your Preferences

Choose activities you like to promote consistency and long-term adherence. Exercise should be a fun and gratifying activity, not a work.

Preferences:

- Activity Enjoyment: Engage in workouts that you find pleasurable, whether it's dancing, hiking, or team sports.
- Variety: Incorporate a diversity of activities to keep your routine fresh and minimize monotony.

2. Evaluate Your Current Fitness Level

2.1. Assess Physical Capabilities

Before starting a new workout plan, analyze your existing fitness level and physical restrictions. Consider elements such as endurance, strength, flexibility, and any pre-existing health concerns.

Assessments:

- Endurance: Measure your capacity to maintain aerobic activity over time.

- Strength: Evaluate your strength with workouts like push-ups or weightlifting.

- Flexibility: Test your range of motion with stretches or flexibility exercises.

- Health issues: Consider any medical issues or injuries that may affect your exercise choices.

2.2. Set Realistic Milestones

Establish attainable benchmarks depending on your fitness level and goals. Setting realistic objectives helps sustain motivation and measure progress.

Milestones:

- Short-Term objectives: Set objectives for the next few weeks or months, such as increasing the number of push-ups or jogging a specific distance.

- Long-Term Goals: Define overall targets, such as running a marathon or attaining a certain weight loss target.

3. Choose a Balanced Exercise Routine

3.1. Incorporate Cardiovascular Exercise

Cardiovascular activities promote heart health, build stamina, and burn calories. Aim for at least 150 minutes of moderate-intensity or 75 minutes of high-intensity aerobic activity every week.

Cardiovascular Activities:

- Walking or Running: Easy to start and may be done inside or outdoors.
- Cycling: Great for increasing lower body strength and endurance.
- Swimming: Low-impact activity that exercises the entire body and promotes cardiovascular health.

3.2. Include Strength Training

Strength exercise enhances muscular growth, boosts metabolism, and promotes joint health. Include resistance workouts targeting key muscle groups at least twice a week.

Strength Training movements:

- Weight Lifting: Use free weights or machines to do movements including squats, deadlifts, and bench presses.

- Bodyweight Exercises: Perform push-ups, lunges, and planks to increase strength without equipment.
- Resistance Bands: Use bands for a range of workouts to develop strength and flexibility.

3.3. Add Flexibility and Balance Work

Incorporating flexibility and balancing exercises boosts range of motion, minimizes injury risk, and improves total functional fitness. Include stretching or flexibility exercises several times a week.

Flexibility and Balance Activities:

- Stretching: Perform static and dynamic stretches to enhance flexibility.
- Yoga: Practice yoga to develop flexibility, balance, and mental focus.
- Pilates: Engage in Pilates to strengthen the core and improve general body alignment.

4. Consider Special Populations

4.1. Adapt for Age and Fitness Level

Modify workout regimens based on age and fitness level to ensure safety and efficacy. Older folks and beginners may require different tactics than younger or more accomplished ones.

Adaptations:

- Older Adults: Focus on low-impact activities, balancing exercises, and strength training with lesser weights.
- Beginners: Start with simple workouts and progressively increase intensity and length.

4.2. Address Health Conditions

Tailor workout regimens to meet any health issues or injuries. Consult with healthcare specialists or fitness experts to build a safe and successful program.

Considerations:

- Chronic diseases: Modify activities to accommodate diseases like arthritis or diabetes.
- Injuries: Avoid workouts that worsen current injuries and focus on rehabilitation exercises.

5. Create a Sustainable Routine

5.1. Establish a Schedule

Develop a consistent fitness regimen that fits with your everyday lifestyle. Aim for a balanced combination of aerobic, strength, and flexibility training throughout the week.

Scheduling Tips:

- Consistency: Set particular days and times for exercises to develop a pattern.
- Flexibility: Allow for adaptations in case of unanticipated changes or obligations.

5.2. Track Progress and Adjust

Monitor your progress and make modifications to your regimen as needed. Track measures like as endurance, strength, and flexibility to assess improvements and create new targets.

Tracking Methods:

- Fitness Apps: Use apps or wearables to monitor workouts and progress.
- Journals: Keep a fitness notebook to record activities, durations, and personal observations.

Choosing the correct exercise program requires analyzing your fitness objectives, evaluating your current fitness level, and selecting a balanced combination of aerobic, strength, and flexibility workouts. By considering personal preferences, adjusting to special populations, and building a sustainable schedule, you may design a workout regimen that promotes your health and well-being. Regularly track progress and make modifications to sustain motivation and continue attaining your fitness objectives.

Benefits of Regular Physical Activity

Regular physical activity is a cornerstone of a healthy lifestyle, giving multiple advantages for physical, mental, and emotional well-being. Engaging in frequent exercise boosts general health, enhances quality of life, and decreases the risk of different chronic diseases. This book discusses the various advantages of regular physical activity and stresses its relevance for sustaining healthy health.

1. Physical Health Benefits

1.1. Cardiovascular Health

Regular physical exercise strengthens the heart and increases circulation, leading to better cardiovascular health. Engaging in aerobic workouts can reduce the risk of heart disease, lower blood pressure, and improve cholesterol levels.

Benefits:

- Heart Function: Enhances the efficiency of the heart, boosting its ability to pump blood.
- Blood Pressure: Helps decrease and regulate blood pressure levels.

- Cholesterol Levels: Increases HDL (good) cholesterol and decreases LDL (bad) cholesterol.

1.2. Weight Management

Physical exercise has a significant function in regulating body weight by burning calories and improving metabolism. Regular exercise helps balance energy expenditure and intake, helping with weight reduction or maintenance.

Benefits:

- Calorie Burning: Increases energy expenditure and assists in weight reduction.
- Metabolism: Boosts metabolic rate, helping to maintain a healthy weight.

1.3. Muscular Strength and Endurance

Strength training and resistance exercises grow muscle mass, improve physical strength, and enhance endurance. This helps to overall functional fitness and supports everyday activities.

Benefits:

- Muscular Growth: Stimulates muscular development and strength.

- Endurance: Enhances the capacity to complete physical tasks and resist weariness.

1.4. Bone Health

Weight-bearing workouts, such as walking or resistance training, build bones and promote bone density. This helps lower the incidence of osteoporosis and fractures.

Benefits:

- Bone Density: Increases bone mass and strength.
- Osteoporosis Prevention: Reduces the chance of bone loss and associated disorders.

1.5. Joint Health and Flexibility

Regular physical exercise helps joint health by preserving flexibility and minimizing stiffness. It also helps avoid injuries by enhancing joint stability and function.

Benefits:

- Flexibility: Enhances range of motion and minimizes joint stiffness.
- Joint Stability: Strengthens muscles around joints, enhancing stability and function.

2. Mental and Emotional Health Benefits

2.1. Stress Reduction

Physical activity is an excellent technique to manage and relieve stress. Exercise causes the production of endorphins, which are natural mood boosters that promote relaxation and well-being.

Benefits:

- Endorphin Release: Boosts mood and decreases symptoms of stress and anxiety.
- Relaxation: Promotes a sense of tranquility and well-being.

2.2. Improved Mood and Mental Health

Regular exercise is related to decreased feelings of sadness and anxiety. Engaging in physical exercise may promote mood, improve self-esteem, and support mental health.

Benefits:

- Mood Enhancement: Elevates mood and lowers symptoms of depression.
- Self-Esteem: Boosts self-confidence and body image.

2.3. Cognitive Function and Memory

Physical activity helps brain health by enhancing cognitive function, memory, and focus. Regular exercise has been related to a decreased risk of cognitive decline and neurodegenerative illnesses.

Benefits:

- Cognitive Enhancement: Improves memory, attention, and learning ability.
- Neuroprotection: Reduces the risk of cognitive decline and dementia.

2.4. Better Sleep Quality

Engaging in regular physical exercise can increase sleep quality and duration. Exercise helps normalize sleep patterns and promotes deeper, more restful sleep.

Benefits:

- Sleep Patterns: Enhances the quality and consistency of sleep.
- Restorative Sleep: Increases the duration of deep sleep periods.

3. Social and Lifestyle Benefits

3.1. Social Interaction

Participating in group sports, fitness courses, or exercise clubs gives chances for social contact and can build a sense of community and belonging.

Benefits:

- Social Connections: Builds connections and stimulates social participation.
- Support Systems: Provides inspiration and encouragement through social networks.

3.2. Increased Energy and Vitality

Regular physical exercise enhances overall energy levels and minimizes symptoms of weariness. Exercise promotes energy and improves everyday functioning and production.

Benefits:

- Energy Levels: Increases overall energy and lowers symptoms of weariness.
- Productivity: Enhances performance in daily duties and activities.

3.3. Enhanced Quality of Life

A consistent exercise regimen adds to a greater quality of life by enhancing physical health, emotional well-being, and overall life satisfaction.

Benefits:

- Life Satisfaction: Promotes a positive perspective and increased general well-being.
- Functional Independence: Supports the capacity to undertake everyday tasks and preserve independence.

4. Disease Prevention and Longevity

4.1. Chronic Disease Prevention

Regular physical exercise helps prevent and control chronic illnesses such as type 2 diabetes, hypertension, and some malignancies. Exercise promotes the body's capacity to control blood sugar, blood pressure, and immunological function.

Benefits:

- Disease Prevention: Reduces the risk of chronic illnesses and disorders.
- Management: Helps manage and reduce symptoms of existing health issues.

4.2. Longevity and Aging

Engaging in regular physical exercise is related to extended longevity and healthy aging. Exercise contributes to preserving functional capacities and minimizing the risk of age-related health concerns.

Benefits:

- Increased Lifespan: Promotes a longer, healthier life.
- Healthy Aging: Supports physical and mental health as persons age.

Regular physical activity gives a wide range of advantages that favorably improve physical, mental, and emotional health. From increasing cardiovascular function and controlling weight to enhancing mood, cognitive function, and general quality of life, exercise is a crucial component of a healthy lifestyle. By adding regular physical exercise into everyday activities, individuals may enjoy the myriad health advantages and lead a more vibrant, full life.

Incorporating Movement into Your Daily Life

Integrating activity into your daily routine is vital for preserving physical health, raising energy levels, and improving general well-being. Incorporating regular physical activity into everyday activities may be both feasible and beneficial, especially for individuals with hectic schedules. This guide gives practical techniques and recommendations for effortlessly introducing activity into all facets of everyday living.

1. Start with a Plan

1.1. Set Realistic Goals

Begin by defining reasonable movement objectives that coincide with your lifestyle and fitness level. Small, incremental goals can lead to sustained improvements and improved health results.

Tips:

- Short-Term Goals: Aim for daily or weekly milestones, such as walking 10,000 steps each day or completing 15 minutes of exercise every day.
- Long-Term Goals: Establish bigger targets, such as raising total activity levels or incorporating various forms of exercise.

1.2. Create a Routine

Develop a regular program for adding activity throughout your day. Consistency helps create habits and ensures that physical exercise becomes a regular part of your schedule.

Tips:

- Daily Integration: Designate certain periods for physical exercise, such as morning stretches or evening walks.
- Flexibility: Adapt your routine to fit varied days and schedules.

2. Utilize Opportunities Throughout the Day

2.1. Active Commuting

Incorporate activity into your commute by walking or cycling to work or taking public transit that requires walking to and from stations.

Tips:

- Walk or Bike: Choose walking or bicycling for short excursions or as part of your regular commute.
- Park Further: Opt for a parking place further away from your destination to increase walking distance.

2.2. Take Movement Breaks

Use pauses throughout your day to indulge in small bursts of physical activity. Stand up, stretch, or undertake brief activities to counterbalance extended sitting.

Tips:

- Stand and Stretch: Perform stretches or mild workouts during work breaks.
- Movement Reminders: Set reminders to move every 30-60 minutes if you work at a desk.

2.3. Household Chores

Turn ordinary home duties into chances for physical activity. Activities like cleaning, gardening, or organizing may be physically engaging.

Tips:

- Active Cleaning: Engage in active cleaning tasks to boost your heart rate.
- Gardening: Use gardening jobs as a method to include strength and flexibility workouts.

3. Incorporate Movement into Leisure Activities

3.1. Active Hobbies

Choose pastimes that entail physical exertion, such as hiking, dancing, or playing sports. Engaging in pleasurable activities helps boost overall mobility and makes training more engaging.

Tips:

- Join Clubs: Participate in local sports leagues, dance courses, or hiking groups.
- Explore New things: Try new things to make exercise interesting and pleasurable.

3.2. Family and Social Activities

Include exercise in social and family events by organizing active trips or games. Activities such as playing tag, going on bike rides, or engaging in family walks improve physical health and togetherness.

Tips:

- Active Outings: Plan outings to parks, trails, or recreational locations that stimulate mobility.
- Family Games: Engage in participatory activities or sports with family and friends.

4. Incorporate Exercise into Your Routine

4.1. Home Workouts

Design and implement a home fitness regimen that matches your schedule and space. Home workouts might include bodyweight exercises, resistance bands, or online fitness programs.

Tips:

- Create an area: Designate an area in your house for exercise and equip it with basic fitness gear.
- Utilize Apps: Use fitness apps or internet videos for guided workouts and diversity.

4.2. Workplace Wellness

Incorporate mobility throughout your work by employing standing desks, conducting walking meetings, or engaging in workplace health initiatives.

Tips:

- Standing Desk: Use a standing desk or adjustable desk to alternate between sitting and standing.
- Walking Meetings: Opt for walking meetings or talks wherever feasible.

5. Embrace Active Lifestyle Choices

5.1. Use Stairs

Choose steps over elevators or escalators wherever feasible. Climbing stairs is an easy approach to boost physical activity and develop your lower body.

Tips:

- Stair Climbing: Incorporate stair climbing into your routine, such as using stairs at work or home.
- Build Up: Gradually increase the number of flights you climb for an extra challenge.

5.2. Incorporate Movement into Leisure Time

Opt for active types of leisure, such as walking or cycling instead of sedentary activities like watching TV. Use your leisure time to indulge in physical activities that you like.

Tips:

- Active Leisure: Choose activities like walking tours or bike rides during leisure time.
- Limit Screen Time: Balance screen time with physical activities.

Incorporating activity into your everyday life may be both practical and gratifying. By setting realistic objectives, exploiting changes throughout the day, and adopting active lifestyle choices, you may optimize your physical health, raise energy levels, and improve overall well-being. Making activity a regular part of your routine not only helps long-term health but also leads to a more active and happier life.

Chapter 5

THE ROLE OF SLEEP IN VITALITY

Understanding Sleep Cycles and Their Impact

Sleep is a basic part of human health that greatly impacts energy, general well-being, and everyday functioning. Understanding sleep cycles and their influence is critical for managing sleep quality and enhancing overall vigor. This chapter discusses the intricacy of sleep cycles, their implications on health, and techniques to increase sleep quality for improved vitality.

1. The Science of Sleep

1.1. Sleep Stages

Sleep consists of numerous phases that cycle during the night. Each stage plays a key role in healing processes and overall health.

Stages:

Non-Rapid Eye Movement (NREM) Sleep:

- Stage 1: The lightest sleep state, moving from awake to sleep. It is a brief phase of relaxation and tiredness.

- Stage 2: A deeper slumber when heart rate decreases and body temperature drops. This stage is critical for memory consolidation and cognitive function.
- Stage 3: Also known as deep or slow-wave sleep, this stage is crucial for physical repair and immunological function.

Rapid Eye Movement (REM) Sleep:

REM Sleep: Characterized by quick eye movements, heightened brain activity, and vivid dreaming. REM sleep is critical for emotional control, learning, and memory consolidation.

1.2. Sleep Cycles

A normal sleep cycle lasts around 90 minutes and includes both NREM and REM sleep. Throughout the night, humans experience many sleep cycles, with greater durations of REM sleep happening in the latter half of the night.

Points:

- Cycle Duration: Each entire sleep cycle lasts roughly 90 minutes, with a normal night including 4-6 cycles.
- Cycle Variation: The proportion of each sleep stage changes throughout cycles, with more deep sleep happening early in the night and increasing REM sleep later.

2. The Impact of Sleep on Vitality

2.1. Physical Health

Adequate and restorative sleep is critical for preserving physical health and vigor. Sleep regulates several physiological functions, including metabolism, cardiovascular health, and immunological function.

Impacts:

- Metabolism: Poor sleep is related to disturbed metabolism and increased risk of weight gain and metabolic diseases.
- Cardiovascular Health: Chronic sleep loss is associated with higher blood pressure, increased risk of heart disease, and stroke.
- Immune Function: Quality sleep supports a healthy immune system, boosting the body's capacity to fight infections and diseases.

2.2. Mental and Cognitive Function

Sleep has a key function in cognitive processes such as memory, learning, and emotional regulation. Insufficient sleep lowers cognitive performance and affects mood stability.

Impacts:

- Memory Consolidation: Sleep improves the consolidation of new knowledge and skills, boosting learning and memory retention.
- Cognitive Performance: Poor sleep reduces attention, problem-solving capabilities, and decision-making ability.
- Emotional Regulation: Adequate sleep improves emotional stability and resilience, lowering the risk of mood disorders such as anxiety and depression.

2.3. Physical Performance and Recovery

Restorative sleep is necessary for physical performance and recuperation. Athletes and active persons benefit from adequate sleep, which assists in muscle recovery and general performance.

Impacts:

- Muscle Recovery: Deep sleep phases stimulate muscle repair and development, boosting sports performance and minimizing injury risk.
- Physical Endurance: Sufficient sleep promotes energy levels, coordination, and general physical endurance.

3. Strategies for Improving Sleep Quality

3.1. Establish a Consistent Sleep Schedule

Maintaining a regular sleep schedule helps regulate the body's internal clock and encourages consistent sleep habits.

Tips:

- Bedtime Routine: Go to bed and wake up at the same time every day, including on weekends.
- Sleep Duration: Aim for 7-9 hours of decent sleep every night, depending on individual needs.

3.2. Create a Sleep-Friendly Environment

A suitable sleep environment fosters greater sleep quality by limiting disruptions and increasing relaxation.

Tips:

- Comfy Bedding: Invest in a comfy mattress and pillows that help healthy sleep.
- Darkness and calm: Use blackout curtains and white noise machines to create a dark, calm sleep environment.
- Room Temperature: Maintain a cool, pleasant room temperature favorable to sleep.

3.3. Adopt Healthy Sleep Habits

Incorporating healthy behaviors into your daily routine will boost sleep quality and overall vitality.

Tips:

- Limit Caffeine and Alcohol: Avoid taking stimulants like caffeine and alcohol close to bedtime, since these might alter sleep patterns.
- Relaxation Techniques: Practice relaxation techniques such as deep breathing, meditation, or moderate yoga before bed to improve relaxation and reduce tension.
- Screen Time Management: Limit exposure to screens and blue light from electronic devices at least an hour before bedtime to prevent interruption to melatonin synthesis.

3.4. Address Sleep Disorders

Seek expert treatment if you encounter chronic sleep issues or signs of sleep disorders such as insomnia, sleep apnea, or restless leg syndrome.

Tips:

- Consult an expert: Consult a healthcare physician or sleep expert for diagnosis and treatment of sleep disturbances.
- Sleep Studies: Undergo sleep tests if recommended to identify and manage particular sleep difficulties.

Understanding sleep cycles and their influence on vitality is critical for enhancing health and well-being. Adequate and restorative sleep enhances physical health, cognitive function, emotional stability, and overall performance. By maintaining a consistent sleep schedule, creating a sleep-friendly atmosphere, adopting good sleep habits, and managing sleep problems, individuals can optimize sleep quality and boost vitality. Prioritizing excellent sleep is a critical component of a comprehensive approach to health and well-being.

Strategies for Improving Sleep Quality

Achieving high-quality sleep is vital for sustaining overall health, well-being, and everyday performance. Implementing successful measures can assist boost sleep quality and promote restorative slumber. This guide gives practical and evidence-based recommendations for increasing sleep quality, ensuring you wake up refreshed and invigorated each day.

1. Establish a Consistent Sleep Schedule

1.1. Set Regular Sleep and Wake Times

Maintaining a consistent sleep pattern helps regulate your body's internal clock, also known as the circadian rhythm. Adhering to regular sleep and wake hours can enhance sleep quality and make falling asleep and waking up simpler.

Tips:

- Fixed Bedtime: Go to bed and wake up at the same hour every day, even on weekends.
- Routine Adjustments: Gradually adapt your routine if needed, aiming for 15-30-minute adjustments at a time.

1.2. Create a Pre-Sleep Routine

Establish a relaxing pre-sleep routine to indicate to your body that it is time to wind down and prepare for slumber. Consistent pre-sleep activities can assist smooth the shift from consciousness to sleep.

Tips:

- Relaxation hobbies: Engage in calming hobbies such as reading, listening to soothing music, or taking a warm bath.

- Wind-Down Time: Allocate at least 30 minutes before bedtime for relaxing and winding down.

2. Create a Sleep-Friendly Environment

2.1. Optimize Bedroom Conditions

Designing a sleep-friendly atmosphere can boost comfort and encourage better sleep. Consider aspects such as light, noise, and temperature to create an optimum sleep atmosphere.

Tips:

- Darkness: Use blackout curtains or an eye mask to keep the room dark and reduce light exposure.
- Noise Reduction: Employ white noise machines, earplugs, or soundproofing measures to decrease bothersome noises.
- Comfortable Bedding: Invest in a high-quality mattress and pillows that give enough support and comfort.

2.2. Maintain a Comfortable Temperature

A cool and pleasant room temperature might encourage better sleep. The ideal temperature for most persons is between 60-67°F (15-19°C).

Tips:

- Thermostat: Adjust your room temperature to keep a cool and pleasant atmosphere.
- Bedding: Use breathable and moisture-wicking mattress fabrics to control temperature.

3. Adopt Healthy Sleep Habits

3.1. Limit Caffeine and Alcohol Intake

Caffeine and alcohol can interfere with sleep quality and change sleep patterns. Reducing or eliminating these drugs, especially close to bedtime, can enhance sleep.

Tips:

- Caffeine Cutoff: Avoid ingesting caffeine-containing beverages (e.g., coffee, tea, energy drinks) at least 6 hours before bedtime.
- Alcohol Moderation: Limit alcohol intake and avoid consuming alcohol within a few hours before bedtime.

3.2. Incorporate Relaxation Techniques

Practicing relaxation techniques can help reduce stress and encourage better sleep. Incorporating these practices into your pre-sleep routine will boost relaxation and preparedness for sleep.

Tips:

- Deep Breathing: Practice deep breathing techniques to soothe the mind and body.
- Meditation and Mindfulness: Engage in meditation or mindfulness activities to reduce anxiety and improve relaxation.

3.3. Manage Screen Time

Exposure to screens and blue light from electronic devices can impair the synthesis of melatonin, a hormone that governs sleep. Reducing screen time before bed can enhance sleep quality.

Tips:

- Screen-Free Time: Limit screen use at least one hour before bedtime.
- Blue Light Filters: Use blue light filters or glasses to limit blue light exposure in the evening.

4. Address Sleep Disorders

4.1. Recognize Signs of Sleep Disorders

Sleep problems such as insomnia, sleep apnea, and restless leg syndrome can dramatically impair sleep quality. Identifying and managing signs of sleep disturbances is vital for improving sleep.

Tips:

- Insomnia Symptoms: Difficulty getting asleep, staying asleep, or waking up too early may suggest insomnia.
- Sleep Apnea Symptoms: Snoring, choking, or gasping during sleep might be indicators of sleep apnea.
- Restless Leg Syndrome: Uncomfortable feelings in the legs that intensify at night may suggest restless leg syndrome.

4.2. Seek Professional Help

Consult a healthcare professional or sleep expert if you encounter recurrent sleep issues or suspect a sleep disorder. Professional examination and therapy can address underlying problems and improve sleep quality.

Tips:

- Sleep tests: Undergo sleep tests or assessments if indicated to identify and treat sleep issues.
- Medical Advice: Follow medical advice and treatment strategies to manage and improve sleep issues.

5. Enhance Daytime Habits

5.1. Increase Physical Activity

Regular physical exercise helps promote improved sleep and general health. Engaging in moderate exercise during the day can help regulate sleep patterns and enhance sleep quality.

Tips:

- Activity Timing: Aim for at least 150 minutes of moderate activity each week, but avoid excessive exercise close to bedtime.
- Daytime exercise: Incorporate physical exercise into your everyday routine, such as walking or exercising during daylight hours.

5.2. Manage Stress and Anxiety

Effective stress management and coping skills can positively improve sleep quality. Addressing stress and anxiety through different strategies can boost general well-being and promote peaceful sleep.

Tips:

- Stress Management: Practice stress-reducing strategies such as yoga, writing, or chatting with a therapist.

- Healthy Coping Strategies: Utilize healthy coping skills to handle daily stress and promote relaxation.

Improving sleep quality includes a combination of maintaining a consistent sleep schedule, developing a sleep-friendly environment, adopting good sleep habits, managing sleep problems, and boosting daily routines. By applying these measures, individuals may boost their sleep quality, promote overall health, and feel more vitality and well-being. Prioritizing sleep as a basic part of health and implementing evidence-based strategies can lead to more restful and restorative sleep.

Overcoming Common Sleep Disorders

Sleep issues can dramatically impair general health, well-being, and everyday functioning. Identifying and managing these issues is vital for getting restful sleep and keeping a high quality of life. This article includes an overview of common sleep disorders, their symptoms, and successful ways of treating and conquering them.

1. Insomnia

1.1. Understanding Insomnia

Insomnia is defined by difficulties getting asleep, remaining asleep, or waking up too early while having ample chance for sleep. It can be acute (short-term) or chronic (long-term) and may stem from stress, anxiety, or other underlying disorders.

Symptoms:

Problems getting asleep or staying asleep - Frequent awakenings during the night - Early morning awakenings and inability to return to sleep - Daytime weariness, irritation, or problems focusing

1.2. Management Strategies

- Cognitive Behavioral Treatment for Insomnia (CBT-I): This evidence-based treatment helps address beliefs and behaviors that contribute to insomnia.
- Sleep Hygiene Practices: Implement proper sleep hygiene, such as keeping a consistent sleep schedule, setting a soothing nighttime ritual, and improving the sleep environment.
- Avoid Stimulants: Limit caffeine and nicotine intake, especially in the afternoon and evening.
- Relaxation Techniques: Practice relaxation techniques such as deep breathing, progressive muscle relaxation, or meditation to reduce stress and encourage better sleep.

2. Sleep Apnea

2.1. Understanding Sleep Apnea

Sleep apnea is a sleep condition characterized by recurrent disruptions in breathing during sleep. The most frequent kind, obstructive sleep apnea (OSA), happens when the muscles at the back of the throat relax excessively, obstructing the airway.

Symptoms:

- Loud snoring
- Choking or gasping during sleep
- Excessive daytime sleepiness
- Morning headaches
- Difficulty concentrating

2.2. Management Strategies

- Continuous Positive Airway Pressure (CPAP): The primary treatment for OSA, CPAP therapy includes wearing a mask that produces continuous air pressure to keep the airway open during sleep.
- Lifestyle Modifications: Maintain a healthy weight, avoid alcohol and sedatives, and sleep on your side instead of your back.

- Medical assessment: Consult a sleep expert for a comprehensive assessment and diagnosis. Treatment may include modifications to CPAP settings or other measures.

3. Restless Legs Syndrome (RLS)

3.1. Understanding Restless Legs Syndrome

Restless Legs Syndrome (RLS) is a syndrome characterized by painful sensations in the legs, coupled with an overwhelming impulse to move them, sometimes worsened in the evening or during rest.

Symptoms:

Uncomfortable feelings in the legs, sometimes characterized as crawling, tingling, or itching - Urge to move the legs to ease discomfort - Symptoms often intensify at night or during periods of inactivity - Relief of symptoms with movement

3.2. Management Strategies

- Lifestyle Changes: Incorporate regular physical exercise, avoid coffee and alcohol, and develop a consistent sleep regimen.
- Iron Supplementation: Low iron levels may contribute to RLS; visit a healthcare practitioner about the need for iron supplementation.

- Medication: In certain circumstances, drugs such as dopaminergic agents, anticonvulsants, or opioids may be administered to control severe symptoms.

4. Narcolepsy

4.1. Understanding Narcolepsy

Narcolepsy is a chronic neurological condition marked by extreme daytime drowsiness, abrupt loss of muscular tone (cataplexy), and interrupted nightly sleep.

Symptoms:

- Excessive daytime tiredness and abrupt sleep episodes
- Cataplexy: Sudden decrease of muscular tone produced by severe emotions
- Hallucinations or vivid hallucinations during sleep onset or awakening - Sleep paralysis: Temporary incapacity to move or talk upon falling asleep or waking

3.2. Management Strategies

- Medication: Stimulants, antidepressants, and other drugs can help control symptoms such as excessive daytime drowsiness and cataplexy.
- Planned Naps: Incorporate brief, planned naps throughout the day to ease excessive tiredness.

- Sleep Hygiene: Follow appropriate sleep hygiene habits to improve overall sleep quality and prevent disturbances.

5. Circadian Rhythm Disorders

5.1. Understanding Circadian Rhythm Disorders

Circadian rhythm abnormalities develop when there is a mismatch between an individual's internal biological clock and the external environment. Examples include delayed sleep phase disorder (DSPD) and shift work disorder.

Symptoms:

- Difficulty falling asleep or getting up at desirable times
- Insomnia or excessive daytime sleepiness - Poor sleep quality and daytime dysfunction

5.2. Management Strategies

- Light Therapy: Exposure to strong light in the morning can assist reset the circadian rhythm and improve sleep patterns.
- Chronotherapy: Gradually altering sleep and waking hours to match with desired schedules might help realign the circadian rhythm.

- Consistent Schedule: Maintain a consistent sleep-wake schedule, including on weekends, to promote a steady circadian rhythm.

Overcoming common sleep problems entails knowing the individual disorder, detecting symptoms, and applying appropriate treatment measures. By addressing underlying reasons, adopting good sleep habits, and seeking appropriate medical assistance when needed, individuals can improve sleep quality and general well-being. Prioritizing sleep health and making proactive efforts to address sleep problems can lead to more restful evenings and a greater quality of life.

Chapter 6

MENTAL AND EMOTIONAL WELL-BEING

The Connection between Mind and Body

The delicate relationship between mental and emotional well-being and physical health is increasingly recognized as vital for total health. The connection between mind and body influences every element of health, from physiological processes to emotional moods. This chapter addresses how mental and emotional health affects physical health and gives ideas for building a holistic approach to well-being.

1. The Interrelationship between Mental and Physical Health

1.1. The Mind-Body Connection

The mind-body link refers to the physiological and psychological interaction between mental moods and physical health. Emotional and mental health may influence physiological functioning and vice versa, producing a dynamic interaction that influences overall health.

Aspects:

- Stress and immunological Function: Chronic stress can compromise immunological function, making the body more prone to disease and infection.

- Mental Health and Chronic diseases: Mental health concerns such as depression and anxiety can aggravate chronic physical diseases including cardiovascular disease, diabetes, and chronic pain.

- Psychosomatic Symptoms: Emotional and psychological elements can appear as physical symptoms, such as headaches, gastrointestinal difficulties, and muscular tension.

1.2. The Role of Neurotransmitters

Neurotransmitters are chemical messengers in the brain that play a significant role in regulating mood, emotions, and body processes. Imbalances in neurotransmitters can influence mental health and physical well-being.

Neurotransmitters:

- Serotonin: Influences mood, sleep, and hunger. Low levels are connected with sadness and anxiety.

- Dopamine: Affects motivation, pleasure, and reward. Imbalances are connected to mood disorders and addictive behaviors.
- Cortisol: A stress hormone that, when continuously increased, can damage different physiological systems and lead to health issues.

2. The Impact of Mental and Emotional Health on Physical Health

2.1. Stress and Physical Health

Chronic stress stimulates the body's stress response system, resulting in physiological changes that might significantly impair physical health. Prolonged exposure to stress might lead to different health complications.

Impacts:

- Cardiovascular Health: Chronic stress can increase blood pressure, heart rate, and the risk of heart disease.
- Digestive Health: Stress can lead to gastrointestinal issues such as irritable bowel syndrome (IBS) and ulcers.
- Musculoskeletal Health: Stress can induce muscular tension and discomfort, contributing to illnesses including tension headaches and back pain.

2.2. Emotional Well-Being and Immune Function

Positive emotional well-being and mental resilience have been demonstrated to support a healthy immune system, whereas negative emotions and mental health disorders can impede immunological function.

Impacts:

- Immune Response: Positive emotions and a strong social support network can increase immune response and lower susceptibility to sickness.
- Inflammation: Chronic stress and negative emotions can promote inflammation, which is associated with several chronic illnesses.

2.3. The Role of Sleep in Mental and Emotional Health

Quality sleep is vital for mental and emotional well-being. Poor sleep can worsen mental health disorders and damage physical health.

Impacts:

- Mood Regulation: Insufficient sleep can lead to irritation, mood fluctuations, and greater vulnerability to mental health illnesses.

- Cognitive Function: Poor sleep impacts cognitive functions such as attention, memory, and problem-solving skills.

3. Strategies for Enhancing Mental and Emotional Well-Being

3.1. Stress Management Techniques

Effective stress management is vital for preserving mental and physical wellness. Various approaches can help decrease and manage stress.

Techniques:

- Mindfulness and Meditation: Practices such as mindfulness meditation can help decrease stress, improve emotional regulation, and boost general well-being.
- Exercise: Regular physical activity has been demonstrated to lower stress, increase mood, and promote mental health.
- Relaxation Techniques: Techniques such as deep breathing, gradual muscle relaxation, and yoga can assist manage stress and promote relaxation.

3.2. Building Resilience and Emotional Regulation

Developing resilience and emotional control skills can increase mental well-being and strengthen coping capacities.

Strategies:

- Cognitive Behavioral Therapy (CBT): CBT helps individuals recognize and improve harmful thinking patterns and behaviors, increasing emotional control.
- Positive Self-Talk: Practice positive self-talk and affirmations to boost self-esteem and regulate negative emotions.
- Social help: Cultivate strong social relationships and seek help from friends, family, or mental health specialists.

3.3. Promoting Mental Health Through Healthy Lifestyle Choices

Adopting healthy lifestyle choices can improve mental and emotional well-being and contribute to overall health.

Choices:

- Balanced Diet: A healthy diet helps brain function and emotional stability. Incorporate a mix of fruits, vegetables, healthy grains, and lean meats.
- Regular Exercise: Engage in regular physical exercise to increase mood, decrease stress, and promote general health.
- Adequate Sleep: Prioritize quality sleep by following appropriate sleep hygiene practices and having a consistent sleep schedule.

3.4. Seeking Professional Help

Professional help is vital for treating mental health disorders and increasing emotional well-being.

Steps:

- Therapy and Counseling: Seek therapy or counseling from qualified mental health specialists to address mental health concerns and create coping mechanisms.
- Medication: Consult with healthcare experts regarding the need for medication to address mental health disorders, if appropriate.
- Support Groups: Participate in support groups or peer networks for shared experiences and emotional support.

The relationship between mental and emotional well-being and physical health is broad and diverse. Understanding this interaction and implementing ways to boost mental and emotional health can lead to greater overall well-being. By managing stress, building resilience, adopting healthy lifestyle choices, and getting professional assistance when required, individuals may cultivate a holistic approach to health that supports both mind and body. Prioritizing mental and emotional well-being is vital for attaining a healthy and meaningful existence.

Techniques for Stress Management

Effective stress management is vital for preserving both mental and physical health. Chronic stress can have harmful consequences on the body, including reduced immunological function, cardiovascular difficulties, and mental health disorders. Implementing several stress management approaches can help lessen these impacts, boost resilience, and promote general well-being. This handbook covers many evidence-based approaches for managing and lowering stress.

1. Mindfulness and Meditation

1.1. Mindfulness

Mindfulness entails paying attention to the current moment without judgment. It can help individuals become more aware of their thoughts, feelings, and bodily sensations, lowering stress and enhancing emotional control.

Techniques:

- Mindful Breathing: Focus on your breath, observing each inhale and exhale. This easy activity might help concentrate your attention and quiet your mind.

- Body Scan: Practice a body scan by directing attention to different sections of your body, recognizing any tension or discomfort, and intentionally relaxing those places.
- Mindful Eating: Pay full attention to the sensory experience of eating, relishing each mouthful and noting the textures and flavors.

1.2. Meditation

Meditation is devoted time for focused mental activities aimed to enhance relaxation and mental clarity.

Techniques:

- Guided Meditation: Use audio guides or applications that give guided meditation sessions focusing on relaxation, stress reduction, or particular goals.
- Loving-Kindness Meditation: Cultivate sentiments of compassion and kindness towards yourself and others via concentrated meditation on positive affirmations and aspirations.
- Visualization: Use visualization techniques to create tranquil and relaxing settings, boosting relaxation and lowering tension.

2. Physical Activity

2.1. Exercise

Regular physical activity is an effective stress management technique. Exercise encourages the release of endorphins, which are natural mood enhancers, and helps lessen the physiological consequences of stress.

Techniques:

- Aerobic Exercise: Engage in activities such as walking, jogging, or cycling to enhance cardiovascular health and lower stress levels.
- Strength Training: Incorporate weight lifting or resistance workouts to increase muscular strength and promote overall physical health.
- Yoga: Practice yoga to integrate physical movement with breath control and awareness, promoting relaxation and stress reduction.

2.2. Movement Breaks

Incorporate small periods of physical exercise throughout the day to fight sedentary behavior and alleviate stress.

Techniques:

- Stretching: Perform brief stretching movements to release muscular tension and increase flexibility.
- Short Walks: Take small walks during work breaks or throughout the day to clear your thoughts and minimize stress.

3. Relaxation Techniques

3.1. Deep Breathing

Deep breathing exercises can trigger the body's relaxation response and minimize the physiological impacts of stress.

Techniques:

- Diaphragmatic Breathing: Breathe deeply from the diaphragm, allowing your abdomen to rise and fall with each breath. This approach improves relaxation and relieves tension.
- 4-7-8 Breathing: Inhale for 4 seconds, hold the breath for 7 seconds, then exhale for 8 seconds. This approach helps quiet the nervous system and create calmness.

3.2. Progressive Muscle Relaxation (PMR)

PMR includes tensing and then progressively releasing distinct muscle groups to reduce physical stress and promote relaxation.

Techniques:

- Systematic Relaxation: Start at the toes and work your way up to the head, tensing and releasing each muscle group for several seconds.
- Body Awareness: Focus on the sensations of tension and relaxation in each muscle area, creating awareness and release of physical stress.

3.3. Autogenic Training

Autogenic training is a relaxation method that involves employing self-suggestions to produce a feeling of calm and relaxation.

Techniques:

- Self-Suggestion: Use positive affirmations and mental images to induce sensations of warmth, heaviness, and relaxation in different places of the body.
- Routine Practice: Incorporate autogenic training into your everyday routine for persistent stress management advantages.

4. Cognitive and Behavioral Strategies

4.1. Cognitive Behavioral Therapy (CBT)

CBT is a therapy method that helps individuals recognize and alter negative thinking patterns and behaviors related to stress.

Techniques:

- Thought Records: Track and assess negative ideas, dispute their validity, and replace them with more balanced and optimistic thoughts.
- Behavioral Activation: Engage in activities that create a sense of achievement or enjoyment, helping to offset stress and boost mood.

4.2. Problem-Solving Skills

Effective problem-solving abilities can assist manage stress by addressing and resolving challenges productively.

Techniques:

- Identify Problems: Clearly identify the stressor or problem producing discomfort.
- Generate Solutions: Brainstorm various solutions and evaluate their viability.

- Implement Solutions: Take practical efforts to solve the situation and lessen stress.

4.3. Time Management

Effective time management can help reduce stress by increasing organization and minimizing emotions of overburden.

Techniques:

- Prioritization: Identify and prioritize activities based on significance and urgency, concentrating on high-priority tasks first.
- Scheduling: Use calendars or planners to arrange chores, establish deadlines, and schedule time for breaks and leisure.

5. Lifestyle Adjustments

5.1. Healthy Eating

A healthy diet enhances general well-being and can help manage stress by supplying important nutrients and balancing blood sugar levels.

Techniques:

- Nutrient-Rich Foods: Incorporate a variety of fruits, vegetables, whole grains, and lean proteins into your diet.

- Regular Meals: Eat frequent meals and snacks to maintain steady blood sugar levels and reduce mood swings.

5.2. Adequate Sleep

Quality sleep is vital for stress management and general wellness. Prioritize sleep hygiene and maintain a consistent sleep habit.

Techniques:

- Sleep Hygiene: Create a tranquil sleep environment, avoid stimulants before bedtime, and keep a regular sleep routine.
- Relaxation Before Bed: Incorporate relaxation strategies such as reading or moderate stretching to wind down before sleep.

5.3. Social Support

Building and sustaining strong social ties can give emotional support and assist manage stress.

Techniques:

- Seek Support: Reach out to friends, relatives, or support groups for encouragement and guidance.
- Build Connections: Engage in social activities and build connections that give pleasant and helpful interactions.

Implementing several stress management practices can help individuals better manage and reduce stress, leading to increased overall well-being. By combining mindfulness and meditation, physical exercise, relaxation methods, cognitive and behavioral tactics, and lifestyle improvements, individuals can strengthen their capacity to manage stress and maintain a balanced and healthy existence. Prioritizing stress management is vital for establishing long-term health and resilience.

Cultivating a Positive Mindset

A positive mentality is vital for attaining personal and professional success, promoting resilience, and boosting general well-being. Cultivating a positive mentality entails adopting attitudes and activities that promote optimism, foster growth, and improve mental and emotional health. This guide discusses the concepts of a positive mentality, practical ways for cultivating it, and the advantages it may bring to all facets of life.

1. Understanding a Positive Mindset

1.1. Definition and Importance

A positive mentality refers to a mental attitude marked by optimism, hopefulness, and a focus on the possibility of growth and accomplishment. It entails perceiving problems as opportunities and having an optimistic mindset, especially in the face of hardship.

Aspects:

- Optimism: Belief in the possibility for positive results and the capacity to overcome challenges.
- Resilience: The capacity to recover swiftly from hardships and adapt to change.
- Growth Mindset: Embracing the belief that talents and intellect can be developed through effort and study.

1.2. Benefits of a Positive Mindset

Adopting a happy outlook can have far-reaching advantages for both mental and physical health.

Benefits:

- Improved Mental Health: Reduced risk of depression, anxiety, and stress.
- Enhanced Problem-Solving: Greater capacity to negotiate problems and discover effective solutions.
- Increased Resilience: Better capacity to withstand setbacks and recover from hardship.
- Enhanced connections: Positive interactions with others, resulting in stronger and more supportive connections.

2. Strategies for Cultivating a Positive Mindset

2.1. Practice Gratitude

Gratitude is recognizing and appreciating the pleasant parts of life. Practicing gratitude helps shift emphasis from negative ideas to pleasant experiences.

Techniques:

- Gratitude Journaling: Regularly write down things you are grateful for to build a sense of gratitude and happiness.
- Express Gratitude: Verbally express appreciation to people for their contributions or generosity, fostering positive relationships.

2.2. Reframe Negative Thoughts

Reframing includes turning negative or unhelpful beliefs into more positive and useful ones.

Techniques:

- Challenge Negative ideas: Identify and examine negative ideas, seeking evidence that contradicts them.
- Replace with Positive Affirmations: Substitute negative ideas with positive affirmations that strengthen confidence and optimism.

2.3. Set Realistic Goals

Setting and attaining realistic objectives creates a sense of success and encourages a good mindset.

Techniques:

- SMART Goals: Set Specific, Measurable, Achievable, Relevant, and Time-bound goals to offer clarity and direction.
- Celebrate Progress: Recognize and celebrate victories, no matter how minor, to sustain motivation and positivity.

2.4. Surround Yourself with Positive Influences

The individuals you interact with may drastically affect your thinking. Surrounding oneself with positive and encouraging persons may increase your attitude.

Techniques:

- Build a Supportive Network: Cultivate relationships with individuals that elevate and inspire you.
- Limit Negative Exposure: Reduce exposure to negative influences, such as pessimistic persons or media sources.

2.5. Practice Self-Compassion

Self-compassion includes treating yourself with love and empathy, especially during tough situations.

Techniques:

- Acknowledge Imperfections: Recognize that everyone makes errors and that imperfection is a natural aspect of life.
- Practice Kind Self-Talk: Replace self-criticism with supportive and encouraging self-talk.

2.6. Engage in Positive Activities

Engaging in activities that generate joy and fulfillment can increase your entire mood and attitude.

Techniques:

- Pursue Hobbies: Engage in activities that you like and that bring a sense of fulfillment and pleasure.
- Volunteer: Helping others via volunteering can create a sense of purpose and enhance sentiments of happiness.

2.7. Maintain a Healthy Lifestyle

Physical well-being substantially influences the mental perspective. Adopting a healthy lifestyle helps foster a good outlook.

Techniques:

- Regular Exercise: Incorporate physical exercise into your routine to increase mood and energy levels.
- Balanced Nutrition: Eat a healthful diet that supports general health and well-being.
- Adequate Sleep: Ensure you obtain adequate quality sleep to maintain cognitive and emotional function.

3. Overcoming Challenges to a Positive Mindset

3.1. Addressing Self-Doubt

Self-doubt may weaken positivism and self-confidence. Addressing it entails identifying and questioning these ideas.

Techniques:

- Reflect on prior victories: Remind yourself of prior achievements and victories to fight self-doubt.
- Seek Feedback: Obtain positive input from others to acquire perspective and strengthen self-confidence.

3.2. Managing Stress and Anxiety

Stress and anxiety may badly affect your thinking. Effective stress management can help sustain positivity.

Techniques:

- Stress-Relief Techniques: Practice relaxation techniques such as mindfulness, meditation, or deep breathing to handle stress.
- Seek Support: Reach out for help from friends, family, or mental health experts when required.

3.3. Navigating Setbacks

Setbacks are a normal aspect of life and can challenge an optimistic mentality. Developing resilience helps manage these obstacles.

Techniques:

- Emphasis on Solutions: Shift emphasis from the problem to potential solutions and activities you can take.
- Learn from Experiences: View setbacks as learning opportunities and utilize them to influence future actions.

Cultivating a positive mentality requires adopting attitudes and practices that enhance optimism, resilience, and overall well-being.

By practicing gratitude, reframing negative thoughts, making realistic objectives, surrounding yourself with good influences, and engaging in positive activities, you may build and maintain a happy mindset. Addressing problems such as self-doubt, stress, and setbacks with appropriate solutions can further enhance a positive mentality. Embracing these approaches may lead to increased mental and emotional health, more personal and professional success, and a more satisfying life.

Chapter 7

BUILDING HEALTHY HABITS

The Science of Habit Formation

Habit development is a key feature of human behavior that affects several areas of life, including health, productivity, and well-being. Understanding the science behind habit development can give significant insights into how habits are created, maintained, and modified. This chapter digs into the mechanics of habit development, investigates the impact of signals, routines, and incentives, and presents suggestions for creating and keeping good habits.

1. Understanding Habit Formation

1.1. What Are Habits?

Habits are habitual actions or patterns that are performed with minimal conscious thinking. They are generated by repeated practice and are triggered by certain stimuli or settings.

Characteristics:

- Automaticity: Habits become automatic over time, requiring less cognitive effort.

- Consistency: Regular repetition in response to particular stimuli fosters habit development.
- Context-Dependency: Habits are generally context-specific, occurring in certain locations or situations.

1.2. The Habit Loop

The habit loop, a notion presented by Charles Duhigg in his book **"The Power of Habit",** is a model that describes how habits are established and maintained. It consists of three components: cue, routine, and reward.

Components:

- Cue: A trigger or signal that begins the habit. It might be internal (e.g., emotions) or external (e.g., time of day, place).
- Routine: The behavior or activity that follows the trigger. This is the habitual response or routine.
- Reward: The favorable consequence or reward that promotes the behavior. It delivers satisfaction or relaxation, deepening the loop.

1.3. The Role of Neuroplasticity

Neuroplasticity refers to the brain's ability to restructure itself by generating new neural connections. Habit development is encouraged by neuroplasticity, whereby repeated activities improve brain circuits linked with certain habits.

Points:

- Strengthening Pathways: Repeatedly practicing a habit improves the brain pathways involved in that activity.
- Automaticity: Over time, the habit becomes increasingly automatic as the brain depends on established pathways.

2. Strategies for Building Healthy Habits

2.1. Setting Clear Goals

Setting clear and measurable objectives is key for successful habit formation. Specific, quantifiable goals give direction and drive.

Techniques:

- SMART Goals: Use the SMART criteria (Specific, Measurable, Achievable, Relevant, Time-bound) to develop clear and actionable goals.
- Sub-objectives: Break major objectives into smaller, attainable sub-goals to sustain motivation and measure progress.

2.2. Identifying Triggers

Identifying and comprehending the signals or triggers that motivate a habit is vital for creating and modifying behaviors.

Techniques:

- Cue Analysis: Observe and evaluate the triggers related to your existing behaviors, including time, place, emotional state, and prior acts.
- Cue Substitution: Replace negative or unhealthy signals with good ones to encourage habit modification.

2.3. Designing Effective Routines

Creating successful and durable routines entails picking habits that are practical and connected with your goals.

Techniques:

- Behavioral Mapping: Map out the ideal routine and identify particular acts to replace existing habits.
- Start Small: Begin with tiny, reasonable modifications to maximize the probability of success and lessen resistance.

2.4. Implementing Rewards

Rewards play a significant role in reinforcing behaviors by giving positive reinforcement and motivation.

Techniques:

- Instant Reward: Incorporate instant, concrete rewards to promote the desired behavior.
- Intrinsic incentives: Focus on intrinsic incentives, such as a sense of success or well-being, to sustain long-term motivation.

2.5. Tracking Progress

Monitoring progress helps preserve motivation and gives insight into the success of habit-building tactics.

Techniques:

- Habit Tracking: Use habit-tracking tools or apps to monitor your progress and celebrate milestones.
- Reflect and Adjust: Regularly analyze your progress and make improvements to strategy as required.

2.6. Building Consistency

Consistency is crucial to habit building. Establishing a routine and keeping consistency in practice improves the habit loop.

Techniques:

- Everyday Practice: Incorporate the habit into your everyday routine to develop consistency and reinforce the behavior.

- Environmental Cues: Use environmental cues, such as visual reminders or prompts, to assist regular practice.

2.7. Leveraging Social Support

Social support can boost motivation and responsibility in habit formation.

Techniques:

- Accountability Partners: Partner with a friend or family member to discuss objectives and measure success together.
- Support Groups: Join support groups or communities with similar aims to obtain encouragement and advice.

3. Overcoming Challenges in Habit Formation

3.1. Addressing Setbacks

Setbacks are a natural aspect of habit building. Addressing them correctly is vital for continuing development.

Techniques:

- Identify Barriers: Analyze and resolve barriers or impediments that limit habit formation.

- Practice Self-Compassion: Treat setbacks with self-compassion and utilize them as learning opportunities rather than reasons to give up.

3.2. Sustaining Motivation

Maintaining motivation over time might be tough. Implement ways to sustain motivation and combat complacency.

Techniques:

- Celebrate Successes: Acknowledge and celebrate successes to reinforce positive behavior and retain motivation.
- Adjust objectives: Modify objectives and routines as needed to keep them relevant and interesting.

3.3. Adapting to Change

Adapting to changes in habit or lifestyle demands flexibility and perseverance.

Techniques:

- Adaptable Planning: Create adaptable plans that can accept changes or disruptions while preserving the fundamental habit.
- Reassess objectives: Reassess and change objectives depending on changing conditions or shifting priorities.

Understanding the science of habit development gives significant insights into how habits are developed and maintained. By harnessing the concepts of the habit loop, neuroplasticity, and effective tactics for setting objectives, detecting triggers, structuring routines, applying incentives, and evaluating progress, individuals may create and sustain good habits. Overcoming hurdles, overcoming failures, and keeping motivated are vital for long-term success. Cultivating healthy habits is a strong tool for boosting well-being, attaining personal objectives, and promoting a happy and productive lifestyle.

Tips for Establishing and Maintaining New Habits

Establishing and keeping new habits is vital for personal growth and attaining long-term success. While forming new habits can be tough, implementing good tactics can boost the probability of success and make the process more manageable. This article includes practical recommendations for forming and keeping new habits, building on ideas from behavioral science and habit formation research.

1. Start Small and Build Gradually

1.1. Begin with Achievable Goals

Starting with modest, manageable objectives helps generate momentum and avoids the chance of being overwhelmed. Small modifications are easy to make and can lead to great progress over time.

Tips:

- Focus on One Habit: Concentrate on building one habit at a time to enhance the probability of success.
- Break Down Goals: Divide huge ambitions into smaller, achievable actions that are attainable and realistic.

1.2. Implement Gradual Changes

Gradually adding new habits into your routine helps for smoother transitions and lessens resistance.

Tips:

- Gradual raise: Start with minimum effort and progressively raise the intensity or length as you get more comfortable.
- Adjust Timing: Integrate the new habit into your old routine at a convenient moment to encourage consistency.

2. Create a Structured Plan

2.1. Set Clear and Specific Goals

Clearly stated goals give direction and incentive, making it simpler to measure progress and stay focused.

Tips:

- Use SMART Criteria: Ensure goals are Specific, Measurable, Achievable, Relevant, and Time-bound.
- Write Down Goals: Document your goals to strengthen commitment and offer a reference point for progress.

2.2. Develop a Routine

Incorporate the new habit into a structured routine to promote consistency and automaticity.

Tips:

- Choose a Trigger: Link the new habit to an existing routine or event to generate a dependable cue (e.g., cleaning teeth after breakfast).
- Create a Schedule: Set set periods for exercising the new habit to build a routine.

3. Use Positive Reinforcement

3.1. Reward Yourself

Positive reinforcement increases the habit loop by linking the new behavior with rewards and satisfaction.

Tips:

- Instant benefits: Provide yourself with instant, concrete benefits for successfully fulfilling the habit.
- Intrinsic incentives: Focus on internal incentives, such as a sense of success or enhanced well-being.

3.2. Track Progress

Monitoring progress helps preserve motivation and offers insight into the success of your methods.

Tips:

- Use a Habit Tracker: Utilize habit-tracking tools or apps to document your progress and celebrate achievements.
- Reflect on Achievements: Regularly examine your progress and appreciate the great adjustments you have achieved.

4. Overcome Obstacles

4.1. Identify and Address Barriers

Understanding and resolving barriers can assist sustain development and prevent setbacks.

Tips:

- Analyze Challenges: Identify possible hurdles to habit development and identify tactics to overcome them.
- Create Contingency Plans: Prepare alternate strategies for dealing with obstacles or disruptions.

4.2. Practice Resilience

Resilience includes being devoted to your goals despite setbacks or obstacles.

Tips:

- Self-Compassion: Treat yourself with care if you meet difficulties and utilize them as learning opportunities.
- Reassess and Adjust: Adapt your strategy as required to meet changes or problems.

5. Leverage Social Support

5.1. Seek Accountability

Accountability partners may give support, encouragement, and incentive.

Tips:

- Find a Partner: Collaborate with a friend, family member, or colleague who shares similar objectives and can give accountability.
- Join a Group: Participate in support groups or communities with common interests to obtain encouragement and advice.

5.2. Share Your Progress

Sharing your success with others helps encourage dedication and provides a feeling of accountability.

Tips:

- Regular Updates: Provide regular updates to your accountability partner or support group to maintain motivation and measure progress.
- Celebrate Successes: Celebrate triumphs and milestones with others to promote positive behavior.

6. Foster a Growth Mindset

6.1. Embrace a Learning Attitude

A growth mindset entails viewing obstacles and failures as opportunities for learning and advancement.

Tips:

- Focus on Growth: Approach habit development with the perspective that abilities and habits can be created through effort and learning.
- Learn from Mistakes: Reflect on any mistakes or setbacks and utilize them to enhance your approach and methods.

6.2. Stay Flexible

Flexibility allows for modifications and alterations, making it simpler to sustain routines under changing conditions.

Tips:

- Adapt objectives: Modify objectives and routines as required to reflect changes in your lifestyle or priorities.
- Be Open to Change: Embrace the necessity for modifications and be open to experimenting with new tactics.

7. Reinforce Positive Habits

7.1. Create Habit Stacking

Habit stacking involves attaching a new habit to an existing one, and employing preexisting routines to support the new behavior.

Tips:

- Choose an Anchor Habit: Select an existing habit that serves as a trigger for the new behavior.
- Build on Success: Start with behaviors that complement and support each other for higher success.

7.2. Maintain Consistency

Consistency is crucial to building and keeping habits. Regular practice helps establish new behaviors.

Tips:

- Daily Practice: Incorporate the habit into your daily routine to establish consistency and encourage automaticity.
- Set Reminders: Use visual or digital cues to urge the new behavior and sustain frequent practice.

Establishing and keeping new habits involves a mix of explicit goal-setting, systematic planning, positive reinforcement, and resilience. By beginning small, building a routine, utilizing social support, and fostering a growth mindset, individuals can boost their capacity to build and sustain healthy behaviors. Overcoming barriers and reinforcing beneficial behaviors lead to long-term success and personal growth. Implementing these principles can lead to substantial and lasting improvements, promoting a healthier and more rewarding living.

Overcoming Barriers to Change

Change is a key component of personal and professional progress, yet it frequently brings major hurdles. Overcoming barriers to change needs a proactive and planned strategy, addressing both internal and external impediments that may impede development. This handbook gives insights into typical hurdles to change and offers practical ways to overcome them.

1. Identifying Common Barriers to Change

1.1. Psychological Barriers

- Fear of Failure: Fear of not succeeding might hinder individuals from seeking change or attempting new techniques.
- Self-Doubt: Lack of confidence in one's ability can hamper efforts to achieve and sustain change.
- Comfort with the Status Quo: A fondness for established routines or habits might produce reluctance to change.

1.2. External Barriers

- Lack of Resources: Insufficient resources, such as time, money, or support, might limit the capacity to seek change.

- Resistance from Others: Opposition or lack of support from coworkers, family, or friends can present difficulties in change.

- Environmental Constraints: External variables such as company culture, rules, or logistical challenges might affect the feasibility of change.

1.3. Organizational Barriers

- Inadequate Leadership Support: Lack of endorsement or support from leaders can weaken reform attempts.

- Poor Communication: Ineffective communication regarding the change process might lead to misconceptions and resistance.

- Unclear Goals or Strategies: Ambiguity regarding the aims or techniques of change can generate confusion and inhibit development.

2. Strategies for Overcoming Psychological Barriers

2.1. Addressing Fear of Failure

- Reframe Failure: View failure as a learning opportunity rather than a setback. Focus on what can be gained from the experience.
- Set Realistic Goals: Break down big goals into smaller, manageable steps to lessen the perceived risk of failure.
- Build a Support Network: Seek encouragement and guidance from mentors, coworkers, or support groups to strengthen confidence.

2.2. Enhancing Self-Confidence

- Recognize talents: Identify and use your talents and prior triumphs to create confidence in your ability.
- Develop Skills: Invest in skill-building and training to develop competence and self-assurance.
- Practice Self-Affirmation: Use positive affirmations and self-talk to promote conviction in your talents.

2.3. Embracing Change

- Acknowledge advantages: Focus on the possible advantages and good consequences of the shift to build a desire to adapt.

- Gradual Transition: Implement change gradually to enable time for adjustment and decrease pain with new habits.
- Engage in Reflective Practices: Reflect on prior experiences with change to recognize successful tactics and approaches.

3. Strategies for Overcoming External Barriers

3.1. Securing Resources

- Conduct a Resource Assessment: Identify and analyze the resources needed for change, including time, money, and support.
- Develop a Resource strategy: Create a strategy to acquire or allocate essential resources, including budgeting and priorities.
- Seek External Support: Explore options for external financing, partnerships, or collaborations to complement resources.

3.2. Gaining Support from Others

- Form partnerships: Engage stakeholders and form partnerships to obtain support and address resistance.
- Communicate Effectively: Clearly express the advantages and reasoning for the change to gather support and understanding.

- Answer Concerns: Listen to and answer concerns or objections from others to develop a collaborative approach to change.

3.3. Navigating Environmental Constraints

- Analyze Constraints: Identify and understand the external elements that affect the feasibility of change.
- Develop Contingency Plans: Create plans to manage potential limits and change strategies as required.
- Argue for Change: Work within current systems to argue for tweaks or modifications that support the change project.

4. Strategies for Overcoming Organizational Barriers

4.1. Securing Leadership Support

- Engage Leaders Early: Involve leaders early in the transformation process to get their endorsement and support.
- Communicate Value: Clearly illustrate the value and benefits of the change to achieve leadership buy-in.
- Foster Collaboration: Collaborate with leaders to build a shared vision and strategy for the change endeavor.

4.2. Improving Communication

- Develop a Communication strategy: Create a complete strategy for communicating the change process, including objectives, dates, and implications.

- Use Multiple Channels: Utilize numerous communication channels to ensure that information reaches all relevant parties.

- Encourage input: Solicit input from stakeholders and address problems to promote understanding and involvement.

4.3. Clarifying Goals and Strategies

- Describe Objectives: Clearly describe the aims and objectives of the change endeavor to offer direction and emphasis.

- Develop a Roadmap: Create a clear roadmap defining the actions, milestones, and resources necessary for effective execution.

- Monitor and alter: Regularly monitor progress and alter techniques as needed to ensure alignment with goals and objectives.

5. Maintaining Momentum and Sustaining Change

5.1. Monitor Progress

- Track Key Metrics: Establish and monitor key performance indicators to measure progress and effectiveness.
- Examine and Reflect: Regularly examine progress and reflect on accomplishments and problems to make informed adjustments.

5.2. Reinforce Commitment

- Celebrate Successes: Acknowledge and celebrate successes and milestones to encourage commitment and drive.
- Maintain Engagement: Keep stakeholders engaged and motivated via frequent updates, acknowledgment, and engagement in the transformation process.
- Adapt and Evolve: Be open to modifying tactics and techniques as needed to handle growing problems and opportunities.

Overcoming barriers to change needs a multidimensional strategy that tackles internal, external, and organizational impediments. By recognizing common barriers, using focused methods, and sustaining momentum, people and organizations may effectively manage the challenges of change. Effective planning, communication, support, and resilience are critical for accomplishing and maintaining significant change, leading to personal and professional growth and success.

Chapter 8

THE IMPACT OF SOCIAL CONNECTIONS

The Role of Community and Relationships in Well-being

Social connections and relationships have a key role in increasing well-being, impacting numerous areas of mental, emotional, and physical health. This chapter analyzes the enormous importance of community and relationships on well-being, giving insights into how social ties contribute to a satisfying and healthy existence.

1. Understanding Social Connections

1.1. The Nature of Social Connections

Types of Social Connections:

- Family: Close-knit ties with family members, including parents, siblings, and extended relatives.
- Friends: Personal ties built through shared interests, experiences, and mutual support.
- Acquaintances: Casual encounters with people you encounter in various circumstances, such as neighbors or colleagues.
- Community: Engagement with larger social networks, including clubs, organizations, and local groups.

Functions of Social Connections:

- Emotional Support: Providing comfort, understanding, and empathy during times of stress or hardship.
- Practical Assistance: Offering aid with everyday duties, problem-solving, and resource sharing.
- Social Interaction: Facilitating chances for socializing, enjoyment, and shared experiences.

1.2. The Science Behind Social Connections

Biological Influences:

- Oxytocin: Often referred to as the "love hormone," oxytocin is released during pleasant social interactions and increases bonding and trust.
- Endorphins: Social contacts can trigger the release of endorphins, which are natural mood boosters.

Psychological Benefits:

- Self-Esteem: Positive social connections contribute to increased self-esteem and a sense of self-worth.
- Cognitive Function: Engaging in social activities can boost cognitive function and mental agility.

2. The Impact of Social Connections on Mental and Emotional Health

2.1. Reducing Stress and Anxiety

Support Systems:

- Emotional Buffer: Having a robust support network may function as a buffer against stress and anxiety.
- Coping tactics: Social relationships offer access to varied coping tactics and viewpoints.

Research Findings:

- Studies: Research has revealed that those with strong social ties have lower levels of stress and are better suited to handle anxiety.

2.2. Enhancing Happiness and Life Satisfaction

Pleasant Interactions:

- Joy and Fulfillment: Engaging in pleasant social interactions and fostering relationships lead to overall happiness and life satisfaction.
- Shared Experiences: Sharing experiences with people develops a sense of belonging and increases life happiness.

Research Findings:

- Studies: Research reveals that persons with supportive social networks report better levels of happiness and life satisfaction.

2.3. Building Resilience

Social Support:

- Resilience: Strong social relationships help to resilience by offering emotional support and practical aid during tough times.
- Encouragement: Supportive connections give encouragement and inspiration to persevere through obstacles.

Research Findings:

- Studies: Evidence shows that persons with robust social support systems are more resilient and better able to recover from adversity.

3. The Impact of Social Connections on Physical Health

3.1. Improving Physical Health

Health Benefits:

- Reduced Risk of Illness: Social ties have been related to a decreased risk of many health issues, including cardiovascular disease and chronic diseases.
- Health Behaviors: Positive social connections can encourage healthy behaviors, such as frequent exercise and healthy eating.

Research Findings:

- Studies: Research has revealed that persons with strong social bonds tend to have better physical health outcomes and longer lifespans.

3.2. Enhancing Longevity

Social Engagement:

- Life Expectancy: Engaging in meaningful social interactions and keeping good connections can lead to an enhanced lifespan.

- Preventative Health: Social connections enhance preventative health activities and early diagnosis of health concerns.

Research Findings:

- Studies: Studies have indicated that those with busy social lives have a decreased chance of death and have longer, healthier lives.

4. Building and Nurturing Social Connections

4.1. Strengthening Existing Relationships

Quality Time:

- Prioritize Relationships: Allocate time for meaningful interactions with family and friends to enhance existing ties.
- Express Appreciation: Regularly express thanks and appreciation to build ties and promote great relationships.

4.2. Expanding Social Networks

Engage in Community Activities:

- Join Groups: Participate in community groups, clubs, or organizations that correspond with your interests and values.

- Attend Events: Attend social events and gatherings to meet new people and grow your social network.

4.3. Developing New Connections

Networking Opportunities:

- Professional Networks: Engage in professional networking opportunities to create relationships with colleagues and industry peers.
- Volunteer Work: Volunteer for causes you care about to connect with like-minded folks and contribute to the community.

4.4. Cultivating Meaningful Relationships

Deepening Connections:

- Authentic Engagement: Foster authentic and meaningful connections by being present, attentive, and compassionate in encounters.
- Active Listening: Practice active listening to understand and connect with people on a deeper level.

5. Overcoming Challenges in Social Connections

5.1. Addressing Social Isolation

Combatting Isolation:

- Seek Support: Reach out to friends, relatives, or support groups if feeling social isolation or loneliness.
- Engage in Activities: Participate in social activities and events to combat isolation and develop new contacts.

5.2. Managing Conflict in Relationships

Conflict Resolution:

- Effective Communication: Use effective communication skills to address and resolve disputes in relationships.
- Seek Mediation: Consider seeking mediation or therapy if disagreements continue or become tough to settle.

5.3. Balancing Social and Personal Needs

Prioritizing Self-Care:

- Set Boundaries: Establish appropriate boundaries to balance social activities with personal time and self-care.
- Monitor Well-being: Regularly analyze and treat your emotional and mental well-being to maintain a healthy balance.

Social ties and relationships greatly affect well-being, impacting mental, emotional, and physical health. Understanding the significance of communities and relationships in promoting pleasure, lowering stress, and improving health helps lead efforts to develop and cultivate meaningful connections. By emphasizing relationships, growing social networks, and addressing issues, individuals may establish a supportive social environment that leads to overall well-being and a satisfying existence.

Strategies for Building Strong Social Networks

Building a strong social network is vital for personal and professional progress. Effective networking may give important assistance, open doors to new possibilities, and boost general well-being. This article covers practical tactics for developing and sustaining powerful social networks.

1. Establishing a Foundation for Networking

1.1. Define Your Networking Goals

Purpose:

- Personal Growth: Identify goals relating to personal growth, such as obtaining new skills or increasing social networks.

- Professional Advancement: Set targets for career growth, such as seeking mentors, investigating employment options, or expanding industry expertise.

Tips:

- Be Specific: Specify what you want to achieve through networking, such as finding a mentor or joining a professional organization.
- Align with Values: Ensure your networking goals coincide with your personal beliefs and interests to develop real relationships.

1.2. Develop a Networking Plan

Planning:

- Identify Key Contacts: List persons or groups that correspond with your aims and interests.
- Set Milestones: Establish clear goals for reaching out to possible connections and attending networking events.

Tips:

- Create a Schedule: Develop a schedule for networking activities, including attending events and following up with connections.

- Track Progress: Use a monitoring system to monitor your networking activities and measure progress toward your goals.

2. Expanding Your Network

2.1. Engage in Networking Events

Types of Events:

- Professional Conferences: Attend industry conferences and seminars to meet peers and leaders in your area.
- Workshops and Seminars: Participate in workshops and seminars to gain information and network with like-minded individuals.
- Social Gatherings: Join social events and gatherings, such as community meetups or alumni events, to broaden your network.

Tips:

- Prepare in Advance: Research attendees and event organizers to find important persons you want to interact with.
- Be Approachable: Use open body language and a welcoming disposition to make a great impression on people.

2.2. Utilize Online Platforms

Platforms:

- LinkedIn: Build a professional profile, connect with industry colleagues, and engage in relevant groups and discussions.

- Social Media: Engage with communities and groups on sites like Facebook, Twitter, and Instagram to connect with individuals who share your interests.

- Professional Forums: Join forums and online communities relating to your field to network with industry pros.

Tips:

- Optimize Your Profile: Ensure your online profiles are full and reflect your abilities and achievements.

- Engage Regularly: Actively participate in online forums and submit quality information to improve your online profile.

3. Nurturing Relationships

3.1. Follow Up and Stay Connected

Follow-Up:

- Write Thank-You letters: After meeting new connections, write individualized thank-you letters or emails to convey your thanks.
- Schedule Follow-Up Meetings: Arrange follow-up meetings or conversations to continue growing the connection and explore additional prospects.

Tips:

- Be Timely: Follow up within a reasonable interval to keep the relationship fresh and relevant.
- Be Genuine: Show genuine interest in the other person's hobbies and achievements.

3.2. Provide Value

Value Addition:

- Share Resources: Offer excellent resources, such as articles, tools, or recommendations, to meet your contacts' requirements.

- Offer Assistance: Be willing to help others with their objectives or obstacles, building a mutually beneficial connection.

Tips:

- Be Proactive: Look for ways to contribute to others' achievement, whether via introductions, advice, or assistance.
- Build Trust: Establish trust by being trustworthy and continually giving value.

4. Leveraging Existing Connections

4.1. Tap into Your Current Network

Utilization:

- Request Introductions: Ask current connections to introduce you to persons who may coincide with your networking aims.
- Leverage Referrals: Seek referrals and recommendations from reliable relationships to broaden your reach.

Tips:

- Be Clear About Your Needs: Communicate your networking goals and the sort of relationships you are seeking with your existing network.
- Show Appreciation: Express thanks to individuals who aid you in developing your network.

4.2. Collaborate and Co-Create

Collaboration:

- Joint Projects: Partner with contacts on projects, initiatives, or events to establish deeper ties and mutual advantages.
- Shared Goals: Work together toward similar goals to develop relationships and boost your network's value.

Tips:

- Identify Synergies: Look for chances where your aims and interests overlap with those of your connections.
- Foster Partnerships: Build collaborative partnerships that give reciprocal advantages and possibilities for advancement.

5. Maintaining and Strengthening Your Network

5.1. Regular Engagement

Engagement:

- Remain in Touch: Regularly check in with contacts to sustain the relationship and remain updated about their activities.
- Share Updates: Keep your network updated on your accomplishments, successes, and changes in your working life.

Tips:

- Use Multiple Channels: Engage with your network through numerous channels, including emails, social media, and in-person meetings.
- Be Consistent: Maintain constant contact to ensure your relationships stay strong and relevant.

5.2. Evaluate and Refine Your Network

Evaluation:

- Assess Relationships: Periodically examine the strength and significance of your network ties.

- Refine Your Approach: Adjust your networking efforts depending on feedback and developing goals.

Tips:

- Prioritize Quality: Focus on developing high-quality relationships that bring reciprocal advantages and support.
- Be Open to Change: Be flexible to change your network and techniques as your personal and professional goals grow.

Building and maintaining a robust social network involves a systematic approach, combining goal-setting, proactive involvement, and relationship nurturing. By increasing your network, utilizing existing connections, and continually delivering value, you may establish meaningful and productive relationships that lead to personal and professional success. Effective networking not only opens doors to new possibilities but also enhances your life with helpful and meaningful contacts.

The Benefits of Positive Social Interactions

Positive social contacts greatly enhance total well-being, including mental, emotional, and physical health. Engaging in meaningful and supportive relationships with others may lead to several advantages that increase quality of life and help personal and professional progress. This handbook covers the different advantages of healthy social connections and their role in promoting a better, more meaningful life.

1. Enhancing Mental Health

1.1. Reducing Stress and Anxiety

Emotional Support:

- Comfort and Reassurance: Positive social interactions give emotional support and reassurance, which can help reduce stress and anxiety.
- Stress Buffer: Supportive connections operate as a buffer against stress, helping individuals manage and cope with life's problems more successfully.

Research Findings:

- Studies: Research reveals that persons with strong social support networks have reduced levels of stress and anxiety, contributing to improved mental health outcomes.

1.2. Boosting Mood and Happiness

Positive Exchanges:

- Joy and laughs: Engaging in fun social activities and sharing laughs with others may considerably increase mood and overall happiness.

- Sense of Belonging: Positive social connections generate a sense of belonging and inclusion, improving emotions of pleasure and well-being.

Research Findings:

- Studies: Evidence suggests that those who routinely encounter pleasant social interactions report higher levels of pleasure and life satisfaction.

1.3. Strengthening Cognitive Function

Mental Stimulation:

- Engaging talks: Meaningful talks and exchanges increase cognitive functions, such as problem-solving and critical thinking.
- Social Learning: Interacting with others exposes individuals to new ideas and viewpoints, fostering intellectual growth and mental agility.

Research Findings:

- Studies: Studies reveal that persons with busy social lives have higher cognitive function and decreased risk of cognitive decline.

2. Improving Emotional Well-being

2.1. Enhancing Self-Esteem and Confidence

Positive comments:

- Validation: Receiving positive comments and encouragement from others enhances self-esteem and confidence.
- Affirmation: Supportive interactions strengthen a sense of self-worth and competence, contributing to a good self-image.

Research Findings:

- Studies: Research demonstrates that persons with supportive social networks have higher self-esteem and more confidence in their talents.

2.2. Providing Emotional Resilience

Support Systems:

- Coping techniques: Positive social connections offer access to varied coping techniques and emotional support during stressful situations.

- Resilience Building: Supportive interactions improve emotional resilience, helping individuals manage and recover from hardship.

Research Findings:

- Studies: Evidence shows that persons with strong social support systems are more resilient and better suited to face emotional issues.

2.3. Fostering Emotional Connection and Empathy

Empathy Development:

- Understanding Others: Positive interactions build empathy by helping individuals comprehend and relate to the feelings and experiences of others.
- Emotional Bonding: Building emotional ties via helpful interactions promotes empathy and creates deeper relationships.

Research Findings:

- Studies: Research shows that beneficial social interactions promote emotional connection and empathy, contributing to more meaningful partnerships.

3. Enhancing Physical Health

3.1. Boosting Immune Function

Health Benefits:

- Decreased Inflammation: Positive social interactions have been related to decreased inflammation and enhanced immunological function.
- Speedier Recovery: Supportive relationships lead to speedier recovery from sickness and surgery by increasing general health and resilience.

Research Findings:

- Studies: Studies have revealed that persons with strong social relationships had superior immune system responses and reduced frequency of sickness.

3.2. Promoting Healthy Behaviors

Healthy Lifestyle:

- Encouragement: Positive social interactions stimulate healthy habits, such as frequent exercise, balanced eating, and adherence to medical recommendations.
- Accountability: Supportive connections give incentive and accountability for keeping healthy lifestyle choices.

Research Findings:

- Studies: Evidence shows that persons with supportive social networks are more likely to participate in healthy activities and maintain a balanced lifestyle.

3.3. Increasing Longevity

Life Expectancy:

- Social Engagement: Engaging in good social interactions has been related to greater longevity and enhanced quality of life.
- Health advantages: The combined advantages of lower stress, increased immune function, and healthier behaviors contribute to a longer, healthier life.

Research Findings:

- Studies: Research reveals that persons with busy social lives and strong social relationships are likely to live longer and enjoy better health outcomes.

4. Building and Maintaining Positive Social Interactions

4.1. Cultivating Meaningful Relationships

Relationship creating:

- Quality Time: Invest time in creating and sustaining meaningful connections via shared experiences and supportive interactions.
- Authentic Engagement: Foster true connections by being present, empathic, and attentive in encounters.

4.2. Practicing Effective Communication

Communication Skills:

- Active Listening: Practice active listening to understand and connect with people on a deeper level.
- Open Expression: Express yourself openly and honestly to develop trust and enhance relationships.

4.3. Engaging in Community and Social Activities

Community Involvement:

- Join Groups: Participate in community groups, clubs, or organizations that correspond with your interests and values.

- Volunteer: Engage in volunteer activities to connect with people and contribute to the community.

4.4. Maintaining a Positive Attitude

Attitude and Behavior:

- Optimism: Approach encounters with an optimistic attitude to generate a supportive and uplifting environment.
- Thankfulness: Practice thankfulness and appreciation in your interactions to boost the quality of your relationships.

Positive social connections give several advantages that boost mental, emotional, and physical well-being. By building supportive connections, engaging in meaningful conversations, and participating in community activities, individuals can enjoy enhanced happiness, less stress, and better overall health. Embracing the advantages of positive social connections adds to a satisfying and balanced existence, boosting personal growth and a better feeling of connection with others.

Chapter 9

HOLISTIC APPROACHES TO VITALITY

Integrating Mindfulness and Meditation

Holistic approaches to vitality focus on supporting the full person—body, mind, and spirit. Among these practices, mindfulness and meditation play a vital role in promoting general well-being. This chapter discusses how integrating mindfulness and meditation into daily life might lead to enhanced vitality, presenting practical tools and insights to help individuals embrace these practices.

1. Understanding Mindfulness and Meditation

1.1. Defining Mindfulness

Concept:

- Current-Moment Awareness: Mindfulness includes maintaining a heightened awareness of the current moment without judgment. It helps individuals to completely engage with their current experiences, thoughts, feelings, and surroundings.

- Acceptance: It stresses accepting one's experiences as they are, rather than seeking to modify or control them.

Benefits:

- Stress Reduction: Mindfulness helps decrease stress by fostering relaxation and a balanced outlook.
- Emotional Regulation: It assists in controlling emotions and boosting emotional resilience.

1.2. Defining Meditation

Concept:

- Focused Attention: Meditation is a technique that includes focusing the mind on a single object, idea, or activity to attain a state of mental clarity and serenity.
- Styles: Common styles of meditation include concentration meditation, mindfulness meditation, and loving-kindness meditation.

Benefits:

- Mental Clarity: Meditation promotes cognitive function and clarity of cognition.
- Emotional Well-being: It adds to emotional stability and a sense of inner serenity.

2. The Benefits of Mindfulness and Meditation for Vitality

2.1. Enhancing Stress Management

Mindfulness:

- Stress Reduction: Mindfulness activities, such as mindful breathing and body scans, can lower the body's stress reaction and promote relaxation.
- Stress Awareness: It raises awareness of stress causes and builds healthier coping methods.

Meditation:

- Relaxation Response: Meditation generates the relaxation response, counteracting the effects of stress and enhancing general well-being.
- Mental Calmness: It helps relax the mind, minimizing the impact of stress on mental health.

2.2. Improving Emotional Health

Mindfulness:

- Emotional Insight: Mindfulness promotes self-awareness and emotional insight, helping individuals to understand and control their emotions more effectively.

- Resilience: It improves emotional resilience by developing a non-reactive, tolerant attitude towards feelings.

Meditation:

- Emotional Balance: Regular meditation practice contributes to emotional balance and stability, lowering symptoms of anxiety and sadness.
- Positive attitude: It creates a positive attitude in life by creating a sense of inner serenity and satisfaction.

2.3. Enhancing Physical Health

Mindfulness:

- Physical Relaxation: Mindfulness techniques contribute to physical relaxation, lowering muscular tension and boosting general health.
- Health Benefits: Research suggests that mindfulness can significantly influence problems such as chronic pain, hypertension, and cardiovascular health.

Meditation:

- Immunological Function: Meditation has been found to increase immunological function, enhancing the body's ability to resist sickness.

- Pain Management: It assists in pain management by modifying the perception of pain and improving tolerance.

3. Integrating Mindfulness and Meditation into Daily Life

3.1. Establishing a Practice Routine

Consistency:

- Everyday Practice: Incorporate mindfulness and meditation into your everyday routine to get their full benefits. Aim for a few minutes each day, gradually increasing the length as you get more comfortable.
- Set a Schedule: Designate certain times for practice, such as in the morning or before bedtime, to build a consistent pattern.

Tips:

- Start Small: Begin with short sessions and progressively increase the exercise as you grow more acclimated to it.
- Create a Space: Set up a calm, pleasant area for your practice to increase attention and relaxation.

3.2. Practicing Mindfulness Throughout the Day

Mindful Activities:

- Mindful dining: Pay attention to the flavor, texture, and scent of your meal, and eat slowly to enhance your dining experience.
- Mindful Walking: Focus on the sensations of walking, such as the movement of your legs and the feeling of the earth beneath your feet.

Tips:

- Be Present: Bring mindfulness to every day activities by remaining completely present and engaged in each moment.
- Use Reminders: Set reminders or signals throughout the day to inspire mindful awareness.

3.3. Exploring Different Meditation Techniques

Techniques:

- Guided Meditation: Use guided meditation apps or CDs to follow along with a structured practice.
- Breath Awareness: Practice breath awareness meditation by concentrating on your breath and monitoring its natural rhythm.

- Loving-Kindness Meditation: Cultivate compassion and kindness towards yourself and others via loving-kindness meditation.

Tips:

- Experiment: Explore numerous meditation techniques to find the ones that connect best with you.
- Be Patient: Allow yourself time to adjust to varied methods and find what works best for your requirements.

4. Overcoming Challenges in Mindfulness and Meditation Practice

4.1. Addressing Common Obstacles

Distractions:

- Mind Wandering: Recognize that it's common for the mind to wander and gently direct it back to concentrate during exercise.
- External Distractions: Minimize external distractions by finding a quiet area and employing tools like earplugs if required.

Tips:

- Acceptance: Accept distractions as part of the exercise and approach them with a non-judgmental attitude.
- Practice Regularly: Consistent practice helps build resistance against distractions and increases attention over time.

4.2. Managing Expectations

Realistic Goals:

- Progress Over Perfection: Focus on progress rather than perfection. Understand that mindfulness and meditation are abilities that develop gradually.
- Short Sessions: Start with short practice sessions and progressively expand the time as you get more comfortable.

Tips:

- Set Achievable objectives: Set realistic and achievable objectives for your practice to retain motivation and develop a sustainable habit.
- Applaud Success: Acknowledge and applaud modest victories and advances in your practice.

5. Measuring the Impact of Mindfulness and Meditation

5.1. Tracking Personal Growth

Journaling:

- Reflect on Changes: Keep a journal to reflect on changes in mood, stress levels, and overall well-being as a consequence of your practice.
- Document Progress: Record any gains in emotional resilience, physical health, and mental clarity.

5.2. Evaluating Well-being

Self-Assessment:

- Regular Check-Ins: Conduct regular self-assessments to measure the influence of mindfulness and meditation on your well-being.
- Seek input: Consider obtaining input from trusted persons or professionals to acquire more insights into your development.

Integrating mindfulness and meditation into daily life offers a comprehensive approach to increasing energy and general well-being. By cultivating present-moment awareness, lowering stress, increasing mental health, and supporting physical health, these activities lead to a more balanced and meaningful existence.

Embracing mindfulness and meditation involves dedication and patience, but the significant advantages they offer make them useful instruments for gaining more vitality and personal growth.

Exploring Alternative Therapies

Alternative therapies comprise a wide range of practices and treatments that are utilized alongside or instead of mainstream medicine. These therapies attempt to improve holistic well-being by treating the physical, emotional, and spiritual elements of health. This article gives an introduction to numerous alternative therapies, their advantages, and concerns for integrating them into your health routine.

1. Overview of Alternative Therapies

1.1. Definition and Scope

Concept:

- Alternative Therapies: These are therapies that are employed as alternatives to standard medical techniques. They frequently focus on natural or non-invasive approaches to boost health and well-being.
- Complementary Therapies: These therapies are used with conventional medicine to enhance general health and increase the effectiveness of existing treatments.

Categories:

- Natural Remedies: Includes herbal medication, essential oils, and nutritional supplements.
- Mind-Body Practices: Encompasses disciplines such as meditation, yoga, and tai chi.
- Physical Therapies: Includes therapies including acupuncture, massage therapy, and chiropractic care.
- Energy Therapies: Involves practices including Reiki, Qigong, and therapeutic touch.

2. Common Alternative Therapies and Their Benefits

2.1. Herbal Medicine

Concept:

- Herbal Remedies: Uses plants and plant extracts for medicinal reasons. Common herbs include ginger, turmeric, and echinacea.

Benefits:

- Anti-Inflammatory: Many herbs contain anti-inflammatory qualities that can assist manage chronic disorders.
- Immune Support: Herbs like echinacea are considered to improve the immune system and prevent sickness.

Considerations:

- Quality and Safety: Ensure that herbal supplements are supplied from reputable suppliers and speak with a healthcare practitioner before usage.

2.2. Acupuncture

Concept:

- Needle Insertion: Involves inserting fine needles into certain locations on the body to enhance energy flow and restore equilibrium.

Benefits:

- Pain Management: Acupuncture is beneficial in addressing many forms of pain, including chronic pain and migraines.
- Stress Relief: It can also help alleviate tension and induce relaxation.

Considerations:

- Qualified Practitioners: Seek therapy from qualified acupuncturists to assure safety and efficacy.

2.3. Chiropractic Care

Concept:

- Spinal Adjustments: Focuses on detecting and treating musculoskeletal diseases using spinal adjustments and manipulations.

Benefits:

- Pain Relief: Effective in reducing back pain, neck pain, and headaches.
- Improved Mobility: Enhances joint function and general mobility.

Considerations:

- Individual Assessment: Consult with a chiropractor to evaluate if this therapy is appropriate for your situation.

2.4. Yoga and Tai Chi

Concept:

- Mind-Body Practices: Both incorporate physical postures, breathing exercises, and meditation to improve physical and mental health.

Benefits:

- Flexibility and Strength: Yoga and tai chi promote flexibility, strength, and balance.
- Stress Reduction: These routines encourage relaxation and mental clarity.

Considerations:

- Instructor Expertise: Participate in lessons conducted by competent teachers to guarantee appropriate technique and safety.

2.5. Reiki and Energy Therapies

Concept:

- Energy Healing: Reiki and other energy therapies entail channeling healing energy to balance the body's energy field and promote healing.

Benefits:

- Emotional Balance: These therapies can assist relieve stress and emotional strain.
- Enhanced Well-being: Promote a sensation of relaxation and overall well-being.

Considerations:

- Personal Belief: The success of energy treatments may depend on personal beliefs and openness to the practice.

3. Integrating Alternative Therapies into Your Health Regimen

3.1. Consultation with Healthcare Providers

Collaboration:

- Discuss with Providers: Consult with your main healthcare physician before commencing any alternative therapies to ensure they complement your present treatments.
- Holistic Approach: Consider combining alternative therapies as part of a complete health plan that includes traditional medical care.

Tips:

- Open Communication: Share your interest in alternative therapies with your healthcare physician and explore any interactions or contraindications.

3.2. Research and Education

Informed Choices:

- Research Therapies: Investigate the advantages, hazards, and evidence supporting various alternative therapies.
- Education: Educate yourself on the procedures and credentials of practitioners to make educated judgments.

Tips:

- Evidence-Based: Seek therapy with scientific evidence supporting their efficacy and safety.

3.3. Personal Experience and Adaptation

Individualization:

- Trial and Error: Be open to trying different therapies to determine what works best for you.
- Monitor Outcomes: Track your progress and analyze the influence of alternative therapies on your health.

Tips:

- Be Patient: Allow time for therapies to show benefits and change your strategy as needed.

4. Addressing Challenges and Considerations

4.1. Safety and Efficacy

Safety:

- Regulation: Choose treatments and practitioners that are regulated and comply with safety guidelines.
- Potential Interactions: Be mindful of potential interactions between alternative treatments and standard drugs.

Tips:

- Consult Professionals: Seek assistance from trained practitioners and healthcare experts to ensure safe and successful usage of alternative treatments.

4.2. Cost and Accessibility

Cost Considerations:

- Expense: Some alternative therapies may not be covered by insurance and can entail additional fees.
- Accessibility: Evaluate the accessibility of treatments and practitioners in your region.

- Budget Planning: Plan your budget and examine the cost issues of integrating alternative therapy into your health routine.

5. Embracing a Holistic Approach

5.1. Balancing Therapies

Integration:

- Holistic Health: Combine alternative therapies with conventional treatments to obtain a balanced approach to health and well-being.
- Lifestyle Factors: Consider lifestyle elements such as nutrition, exercise, and stress management as part of your holistic health strategy.

Tips:

- Personalized Plan: Develop a personalized health plan that integrates a range of therapies and behaviors to boost overall vitality.

5.2. Continuous Learning and Adaptation

Learning:

- Stay Informed: Keep up-to-date with breakthroughs in alternative therapies and developing research.
- Change Practices: Continuously change your approach depending on personal experiences and emerging evidence.

Tips:

- Open mentality: Maintain an open and curious mentality to investigate new therapies and practices that may increase your well-being.

Exploring alternative therapies gives a significant chance to promote general health and well-being through a holistic approach. By learning the benefits and considerations of various therapies, incorporating them deliberately into your health routine, and addressing any problems, you can construct a holistic and individualized approach to vitality. Embracing alternative therapies with educated decisions and a balanced viewpoint leads to a happier and healthier existence.

The Benefits of a Holistic Health Approach

A holistic health approach stresses the interconnection of body, mind, and spirit, trying to enhance total well-being rather than only addressing individual symptoms or disorders. This holistic view analyzes numerous elements of health and well-being, understanding that physical, emotional, mental, and spiritual variables are profoundly interrelated. This article covers the multiple benefits of adopting a holistic health approach and how it may contribute to a more balanced and fulfilled existence.

1. Comprehensive Well-being

1.1. Addressing the Whole Person

Holistic Perspective:

- Integrated Health: A holistic approach addresses not just physical symptoms but also emotional, mental, and spiritual elements of health.
- Personalized Care: It respects the uniqueness of each individual and tailors health interventions to match their distinctive needs and preferences.

Benefits:

- Balanced Health: By addressing all elements of health, individuals feel a more balanced and integrated sense of well-being.
- Enhanced Quality of Life: A holistic approach enhances overall quality of life by encouraging harmony and balance in all areas of health.

1.2. Preventative Focus

Proactive Measures:

- Early Detection: Holistic health emphasizes preventative care and early detection of possible illnesses before they evolve into more serious conditions.
- Lifestyle Optimization: It emphasizes healthy lifestyle behaviors, such as adequate eating, frequent exercise, and stress management, to avoid sickness and preserve well-being.

Benefits:

- Reduced Health Risks: Proactive measures and preventative treatment lower the risk of chronic illnesses and health issues.

- Long-term Health: By concentrating on prevention, individuals can experience better long-term health outcomes and a higher quality of life.

2. Improved Emotional and Mental Health

2.1. Enhanced Emotional Resilience

Mind-Body Connection:

- Emotional Awareness: A holistic approach improves emotional awareness and gives tools for regulating emotions successfully.
- Stress Reduction: Techniques such as mindfulness, meditation, and relaxation exercises can decrease stress and improve emotional resilience.

Benefits:

- Emotional Stability: Improved emotional resilience leads to improved emotional stability and a more optimistic attitude in life.
- Reduced Anxiety and despair: Holistic practices can help ease feelings of anxiety and despair, contributing to greater mental health.

2.2. Greater Mental Clarity

Cognitive Health:

- Mindfulness techniques: Holistic methods generally incorporate mindfulness and cognitive techniques that increase mental clarity and attention.
- Balanced Lifestyle: By addressing many elements of health, individuals enjoy increased cognitive performance and mental sharpness.

Benefits:

- Improved Focus: Enhanced mental clarity leads to enhanced focus, decision-making, and problem-solving abilities.
- Cognitive Resilience: A comprehensive approach improves cognitive health and resilience, minimizing the risk of cognitive decline.

3. Enhanced Physical Health

3.1. Holistic Physical Care

Integrated Health Practices:

- Complementary treatments: A holistic approach typically incorporates complementary treatments, such as acupuncture, chiropractic care, and herbal medicine, which can assist physical health and recovery.

- Balanced Nutrition: Emphasizes a balanced diet that supports overall health and addresses nutritional demands.

Benefits:

- Improved Health results: Integrated health practices and a balanced diet contribute to enhanced physical health results and overall vigor.

- Faster Recovery: Complementary treatments and proper eating can promote recovery from disease and injuries.

3.2. Greater Physical Resilience

Lifestyle Factors:

- Exercise and exercise: A comprehensive approach emphasizes regular physical exercise, which increases physical resilience and boosts general well-being.

- Good behaviors: Emphasizes the formation of good behaviors that contribute to physical health and lifespan.

Benefits:

- Enhanced Vitality: Regular exercise and good habits enhance physical vitality and energy levels.

- Enhanced lifespan: Adopting a holistic approach to physical health can lead to an enhanced lifespan and a more active lifestyle.

4. Strengthened Spiritual Well-being

4.1. Spiritual Connection

Inner Fulfillment:

- Spiritual activities: A holistic approach may incorporate spiritual activities such as meditation, prayer, or introspection, which create inner fulfillment and a sense of purpose.
- Personal Growth: Encourages personal growth and self-discovery, leading to a better knowledge of one's values and views.

Benefits:

- Inner calm: Spiritual activities lead to a sense of inner calm and happiness, boosting general well-being.
- Purpose and Meaning: Strengthening spiritual connection creates a feeling of purpose and meaning in life.

4.2. Holistic Balance

Integrated Approach:

- Harmony: A holistic approach creates harmony between the physical, emotional, mental, and spiritual elements of health.
- Living Integration: Encourages integrating holistic practices into daily living, producing a balanced and meaningful lifestyle.

Benefits:

- Comprehensive Well-being: Achieving balance in all aspects of health leads to a more harmonious and comprehensive feeling of well-being.
- Fulfilled Life: A balanced approach to health creates a more meaningful and pleasant life experience.

5. Practical Considerations for Adopting a Holistic Health Approach

5.1. Setting Goals and Priorities

Health Planning:

- Define Objectives: Set precise health and wellness objectives that represent your particular requirements and priorities.

- Create a Plan: Develop a comprehensive health plan that encompasses physical, emotional, mental, and spiritual disciplines.

Tips:

- Personalized Approach: Tailor your health plan to match your specific requirements and preferences.
- Regular Evaluation: Regularly analyze and adapt your health plan depending on your progress and growing requirements.

5.2. Seeking Professional Guidance

Expert Consultation:

- Holistic Practitioners: Consult with experienced holistic health practitioners to gain direction and help in adopting a holistic approach.
- Healthcare Integration: Work with your primary healthcare practitioner to blend holistic approaches with traditional medical care.

Tips:

- Qualified Practitioners: Choose practitioners with necessary certificates and experience.

- Collaborative Care: Foster collaboration between holistic practitioners and traditional healthcare specialists for complete care.

A holistic health approach offers multiple benefits by treating the interrelated areas of body, mind, and spirit. By concentrating on overall well-being, better emotional and mental health, increased physical health, and heightened spiritual satisfaction, individuals may attain a more balanced and meaningful existence. Adopting a holistic approach requires defining clear goals, getting expert assistance, and integrating numerous activities into everyday life to improve total vitality and well-being. Embracing this complete perspective fosters a peaceful and enriched life experience.

Chapter 10

PERSONALIZING YOUR HEALTH JOURNEY

Assessing Your Unique Energy Needs

Personalizing your health journey requires knowing and treating your particular energy demands to enhance overall well-being. Each person has specific physical, emotional, and mental requirements that impact their energy levels and health results. This chapter covers ways to analyze your energy demands and presents practical solutions to modify your health practices to promote your vitality.

1. Understanding Your Energy Profile

1.1. Defining Energy Needs

Concept:

- Individual Energy Requirements: Energy demands vary depending on factors such as age, lifestyle, health state, and personal ambitions.
- Energy Balance: Maintaining a balance between energy intake and expenditure is vital for general health and well-being.

Assessment:

- Self-Assessment: Reflect on your everyday energy levels, recognizing patterns of weariness, motivation, and general vitality.
- Health Evaluation: Consider how your physical, emotional, and mental health state influences your energy levels.

1.2. Identifying Key Factors

Physical Factors:

- Diet and Nutrition: Assess how your food choices affect your energy levels and general health.
- Sleep Quality: Evaluate your sleep habits and their influence on your energy and everyday functioning.

Emotional and Mental Factors:

- Stress Levels: Identify causes of stress and their influence on your energy levels and emotional well-being.
- Mental Health: Consider how mental health disorders, such as anxiety or depression, impact your energy and vitality.

2. Methods for Assessing Energy Needs

2.1. Self-Monitoring and Reflection

Journaling:

- Daily Logs: Keep a daily diary to chronicle your energy levels, nutritional intake, physical activity, sleep patterns, and emotional condition.
- Patterns and Trends: Analyze the journal to uncover patterns or trends connected to changes in energy and general well-being.

Tools:

- Energy Tracking Apps: Use smartphone applications developed for measuring energy levels, sleep quality, and physical activity to acquire insights into your energy demands.

2.2. Professional Assessments

Health Screenings:

- Medical Evaluations: Schedule frequent check-ups and health screenings to examine physical health and detect any underlying disorders influencing your energy.

- Nutritional evaluations: Consult with a trained dietitian or nutritionist for individualized dietary evaluations and recommendations.

Mental Health Evaluations:

- Therapeutic Assessment: Work with a mental health expert to analyze emotional and psychological variables influencing your energy and well-being.
- Stress Management: Seek help on appropriate stress management practices to increase energy levels.

3. Tailoring Your Health Practices

3.1. Optimizing Nutrition

Personalized Diet:

- Balanced Meals: Develop a meal plan that incorporates a balance of macronutrients (proteins, carbs, and fats) and micronutrients to maintain sustained energy levels.
- Specialized Diets: Consider any unique dietary demands or limits based on health problems or personal objectives.

Nutritional Adjustments:

- Energy-Boosting Foods: Incorporate foods renowned for their energy-boosting characteristics, such as whole grains, lean meats, fruits, and vegetables.
- Hydration: Ensure appropriate hydration by drinking sufficient water and including hydrating items in your diet.

3.2. Enhancing Sleep Quality

Sleep Optimization:

- Sleep Hygiene: Implement appropriate sleep hygiene habits, such as keeping a consistent sleep schedule, generating a tranquil sleep environment, and avoiding stimulants before bedtime.
- Sleep Assessment: Monitor your sleep habits and make modifications to enhance the quality and length of your sleep.

Tools:

- Sleep Trackers: Use sleep monitoring devices or applications to monitor sleep quality and uncover variables impacting your slumber.

3.3. Managing Stress and Emotional Well-being

Stress Reduction methods:

- Mindfulness and Relaxation: Incorporate mindfulness practices, relaxation methods, and stress management strategies to decrease stress and enhance emotional resilience.
- Therapeutic Support: Engage in therapy or counseling to address emotional difficulties and increase mental well-being.

Emotional Self-Care:

- Support Systems: Build and sustain supportive relationships and social ties that contribute to emotional well-being.
- Self-Care Practices: Prioritize self-care activities that promote relaxation and emotional equilibrium.

4. Setting Goals and Monitoring Progress

4.1. Goal Setting

Personal Objectives:

- Specific Goals: Set precise, measurable, attainable, relevant, and time-bound (SMART) goals relating to boosting energy levels and general well-being.
- Action Plan: Develop an action plan that contains strategies for reaching your goals and implementing individualized health habits.

4.2. Progress Evaluation

Regular Check-Ins:

- Self-Assessment: Regularly examine your progress toward your objectives and make improvements to your health practices as appropriate.
- Input and Adjustment: Seek input from healthcare professionals or wellness coaches to adjust your strategy and boost results.

Tools:

- Progress Tracking: Use journals, apps, or progress charts to monitor improvements and indicate areas needing future focus.

5. Adapting to Changes

5.1. Flexibility and Adaptation

Living Changes:

- Health Changes: Adapt your health habits in response to changes in your health condition or living circumstances.
- Evolving demands: Reassess and alter your strategy as your energy demands and personal goals grow over time.

5.2. Continuous Learning

Staying educated:

- Education: Stay educated on new studies, trends, and practices relevant to energy and well-being.
- Adaptation: Be open to embracing new strategies or making modifications to better your health journey.

Assessing your specific energy demands is a vital step in tailoring your health journey and boosting overall well-being. By recognizing your requirements, adopting effective evaluation techniques, and adjusting health routines to match your personal needs, you may attain a more balanced and invigorated existence. Regular review, goal planning, and adaptation are crucial to sustaining success and addressing any changes in your health or lifestyle. Embracing a tailored approach fosters prolonged energy and a fulfilling health journey.

Creating a Personalized Health Plan

A personalized health plan is a specific approach developed to fit your particular health requirements and goals. It blends multiple areas of well-being, including diet, physical exercise, mental well-being, and lifestyle adjustments, to improve overall health and vitality. This book describes the steps to construct a successful personalized health plan that matches your particular requirements and promotes your long-term well-being.

1. Assessing Your Current Health Status

1.1. Comprehensive Health Evaluation

Health Assessment:

- Medical Check-Up: Begin with a full medical assessment to analyze your current health state, detect any underlying issues, and examine your medical history.

- Diagnostic Tests: Utilize relevant diagnostic tests and screenings to acquire insights into your physical health and find areas for improvement.

Lifestyle Review:

- Diet and Nutrition: Analyze your present eating habits, nutritional consumption, and any dietary limitations or preferences.
- Physical Activity: Evaluate your level of physical activity, including the kind, frequency, and intensity of exercise.
- Sleep Patterns: Assess your sleep quality, length, and any concerns influencing your rest.

Mental and Emotional Health:

- Emotional Well-being: Reflect on your emotional state, stress levels, and mental health issues that may affect your overall health.
- Stress Factors: Identify sources of stress and coping techniques presently in use.

2. Setting Health Goals

2.1. Defining Objectives

SMART Goals:

- Specific: Identify your health targets (e.g., "Increase physical activity to 150 minutes per week").
- Measurable: Establish criteria to monitor success (e.g., "Track daily calorie intake using a mobile app").
- Achievable: Set reasonable and attainable objectives based on your present health state and resources.
- Relevant: Ensure goals correspond with your overall health priorities and personal beliefs.
- Time-Bound: Set a schedule for reaching your goals (e.g., "Achieve target weight in six months").

2.2. Prioritizing Goals

Focus Areas:

- Immediate Needs: Address acute health issues or situations that demand immediate treatment.
- Long-Term Aspirations: Include long-term objectives relating to general well-being and quality of life.

Tips:

- Balance Goals: Create a balanced strategy that contains a combination of short-term and long-term goals to ensure ongoing success.

3. Developing Your Health Plan

3.1. Nutritional Planning

Dietary Adjustments:

- Meal Planning: Develop a meal plan that contains a range of nutrient-dense meals to fulfill your dietary needs and support your health objectives.
- Portion Control: Implement portion control measures to limit calorie intake and encourage healthy eating habits.

Special Considerations:

- Allergies and Intolerances: Account for any food allergies or intolerances in your dietary plan.
- Lifestyle Preferences: Incorporate dietary choices or constraints, such as vegetarian or vegan diets.

3.2. Physical Activity

Exercise Routine:

- Activity Type: Select physical activities that you love and are suited for your fitness level (e.g., walking, cycling, strength training).
- Frequency and Duration: Establish a regular workout plan with adequate frequency and duration to reach your fitness objectives.

Tips:

- Variety: Include a combination of cardiovascular, strength, and flexibility exercises to achieve a well-rounded fitness regimen.

3.3. Sleep and Rest

Sleep Hygiene:

- Sleep routine: Create a regular sleep routine with consistent bedtimes and wake-up timings.
- Sleep Environment: Optimize your sleep environment by keeping a pleasant and quiet setting conducive to peaceful sleep.

Rest and recuperation:

- Rest Days: Incorporate rest days into your physical activity program to allow for recuperation and prevent overexertion.
- Relaxation Techniques: Practice relaxation techniques such as deep breathing, meditation, or progressive muscle relaxation to enhance sleep quality.

3.4. Mental and Emotional Well-being

Stress Management:

- Stress Reduction: Integrate stress management strategies such as mindfulness, yoga, or journaling into your daily routine.
- Emotional help: Seek help from mental health specialists, if needed, to address any emotional or psychological difficulties.

Self-Care:

- Personal Time: Allocate time for self-care activities that encourage relaxation and emotional equilibrium.
- Social ties: Maintain healthy relationships and social ties to improve emotional well-being.

4. Implementing Your Plan

4.1. Action Steps

Daily Routine:

- Daily Practices: Incorporate your health plan aspects into your daily routine, including food, exercise, sleep, and self-care activities.
- Consistency: Aim for consistency in following your health plan to attain the greatest outcomes.

4.2. Monitoring and Adjusting

Monitoring Progress:

- Regular Check-Ins: Monitor your progress towards your objectives by monitoring relevant indicators, such as weight, fitness levels, or sleep quality.
- Feedback and Adjustment: Review your progress occasionally and make adjustments to your plan as needed to meet any problems or changes in your health.

Tips:

- Stay Flexible: Be flexible to altering your strategy depending on feedback and growing health requirements.

5. Seeking Professional Guidance

5.1. Expert Consultation

Healthcare Providers:

- Medical Advice: Consult with healthcare providers, such as physicians, dietitians, and fitness experts, for tailored advice and guidance.
- Specialist help: Seek specialist help if you have unique health conditions or goals that require professional involvement.

5.2. Collaborative Care

Integration:

- Holistic Approach: Collaborate with healthcare providers to combine your individualized health plan with traditional medical care and other therapeutic approaches.
- Coordination: Ensure that all components of your health plan are coordinated to ensure complete and effective results.

Creating a personalized health plan entails a comprehensive assessment of your current health state, identifying clear and realistic goals, and designing a specialized approach to suit your requirements. By adding components such as diet, physical exercise, sleep, and mental well-being into your plan, you may enhance your overall health and vitality. Regular monitoring, correction, and expert advice are vital to maintaining development and attaining long-term success. Embracing a tailored approach encourages a happier, more balanced existence and allows you to take care of your well-being.

Monitoring Progress and Adjusting Strategies

Monitoring progress and changing techniques are critical components of a successful personalized health plan. Regularly monitoring your progress helps verify that your health goals are being fulfilled and enables for timely changes to maximize outcomes. This article covers efficient strategies for measuring your progress, finding areas for improvement, and making appropriate modifications to your health plan.

1. Tracking Progress

1.1. Setting Metrics and Indicators

Objective Measurement:

- Health Metrics: Define particular metrics to evaluate progress, such as weight, body measurements, fitness levels, blood pressure, or cholesterol levels.

- Activity records: Use activity records to track physical exercise, nutritional consumption, and sleep habits.

Tools and Resources:

- Tracking applications: Utilize mobile applications and wearable devices to measure metrics like as daily steps, calorie consumption, and sleep quality.
- Journals: Maintain a health diary to document daily activities, emotions, and any symptoms or changes in your condition.

1.2. Regular Check-Ins

Routine Evaluation:

- Weekly or Monthly Reviews: Schedule frequent intervals to monitor your progress against defined goals (e.g., weekly, bi-weekly, or monthly).
- Self-Assessment: Conduct self-assessments to evaluate how well you are sticking to your health plan and highlight any obstacles or triumphs.

Professional Assessments:

- Healthcare Visits: Schedule frequent consultations with healthcare providers to measure physical health indicators and obtain professional comments.

- Progress Reports: Request progress updates from fitness trainers, nutritionists, or other experts involved with your treatment.

2. Identifying Areas for Improvement

2.1. Analyzing Results

Performance Evaluation:

- Goal Achievement: Compare your actual outcomes with your health objectives to evaluate if you are on track or falling short.
- Trend Analysis: Analyze trends in your data to detect patterns or concerns that may hinder your development (e.g., variations in energy levels or uneven sleep quality).

Feedback Collection:

- Self-Reflection: Reflect on your experiences and struggles to identify any roadblocks or impediments impeding your development.
- Professional Input: Seek comments from healthcare experts or wellness coaches to acquire insights into areas needing improvement.

2.2. Addressing Challenges

Problem Identification:

- Obstacles: Identify particular obstacles or issues that have slowed your development, such as nutritional challenges, lack of enthusiasm, or schedule conflicts.
- Root Causes: Determine the root causes of these difficulties to solve them effectively.

Solutions and Strategies:

- Adjustments: Modify your health plan to meet recognized issues, such as altering nutritional consumption, changing exercise routines, or adding stress management approaches.
- Support Systems: Enhance your support systems by accessing extra resources or expert guidance if needed.

3. Adjusting Strategies

3.1. Making Modifications

Plan Refinement:

- Goal Adjustment: Modify your health objectives as required depending on progress, changes in health status, or developing priorities.

- Strategy Changes: Adjust tactics relating to diet, exercise, sleep, or mental well-being to better correspond with your requirements and objectives.

Practical Adjustments:

- Dietary Changes: Revise your meal plan to accommodate new foods, change portion sizes, or meet particular nutritional needs.
- Exercise regimen: Modify your exercise regimen to incorporate various types of activity, increase intensity, or modify frequency.

3.2. Implementing New Approaches

Innovative Practices:

- New Techniques: Explore new techniques or practices that may boost your health plan, such as attempting new workout methods or adding relaxation activities.
- Alternative Therapies: Consider incorporating alternative therapies, such as acupuncture or massage, if they correspond with your health objectives and requirements.

Lifestyle Integration:

- Behavioral modifications: Implement behavioral modifications to increase adherence to your health plan, such as setting reminders, forming routines, or building new habits.

- Environmental Modifications: Make adjustments to your surroundings that complement your health objectives, such as organizing an exercise area or stocking up on healthy meals.

4. Staying Motivated and Committed

4.1. Goal Reaffirmation

Revisiting Objectives:

- Goal Review: Periodically revisit your objectives to reinforce their relevance and importance.

- Success Acknowledgment: Celebrate successes and milestones to sustain motivation and acknowledge your development.

4.2. Maintaining Engagement

Motivational Strategies:

- Accountability Partners: Engage with accountability partners, such as friends, family members, or support groups, to stay motivated and committed.
- Incentives and prizes: Set up incentives and prizes for hitting specified milestones or keeping consistency in your health plan.

4.3. Flexibility and Adaptation

Adaptation:

- Open-Minded Approach: Stay open to altering your health plan as required depending on progress, feedback, and changing circumstances.
- Continuous Improvement: Embrace a philosophy of continuous improvement, exploring methods to increase your health and well-being throughout time.

Monitoring progress and changing techniques are vital for the efficacy of your individualized health plan. By measuring important indicators, reviewing results, resolving difficulties, and making required revisions, you can guarantee that your health plan remains aligned with your goals and developing requirements.

Staying motivated and dedicated, while keeping flexibility, enables sustained development and long-term success in reaching maximum health and vitality. Regular reviews and smart modifications enable you to take control of your health journey and attain a balanced and meaningful life.

Chapter 11

SUSTAINABLE LIVING FOR LONG-TERM VITALITY

Adopting Eco-friendly Practices

Embracing sustainable living is key to boosting long-term vitality and well-being. Eco-friendly methods not only benefit the environment but also contribute to a healthier lifestyle by decreasing exposure to chemicals and fostering mindful living. This chapter discusses the significance of sustainable living, practical strategies to adopt eco-friendly activities, and the good impact these changes may have on your health and the globe.

1. Understanding Sustainable Living

1.1. Definition and Importance

Sustainable Living:

Sustainable living entails making decisions that limit your environmental effects and improve the well-being of the world.

Importance

Adopting sustainable practices helps conserve natural resources, decrease pollution, and create a better environment for future generations.

Health Benefits:

- Reduced Toxins: Eco-friendly goods and activities decrease exposure to dangerous chemicals and pollutants.
- Enhanced Well-being: Sustainable living creates a connection to nature, supporting physical and mental health.

1.2. The Connection to Vitality

Environmental Impact on Health:

- Clean Air and Water: Reducing pollution improves air and water quality, which directly influences respiratory and general health.
- Nutritious Food: Sustainable agriculture techniques guarantee the availability of fresh, nutrient-dense foods, supporting healthy nutrition and energy levels.

Holistic Approach:

- Mindful Living: Adopting sustainable habits fosters awareness and a sense of responsibility toward the environment, boosting mental and emotional well-being.

2. Practical Ways to Adopt Eco-friendly Practices

2.1. Sustainable Consumption

Eco-friendly goods:

- Natural and Organic: Choose natural, organic, and non-toxic goods for personal care, cleaning, and home usage.
- Reusable Items: Opt for reusable products such as water bottles, shopping bags, and food containers to decrease waste.

Conscious Shopping:

- Local and Ethical: Support local companies and ethical brands that value sustainability and fair trade methods.
- Minimalism: Practice minimalism by acquiring only what you need and concentrating on quality over quantity.

2.2. Reducing Waste

Trash Management:

- Recycling: Recycle paper, plastic, glass, and metal products to decrease landfill trash.
- Composting: Compost organic waste to generate nutrient-rich soil for gardening and decrease food waste.

Zero-Waste Lifestyle:

- Packaging: Choose items with minimum or recyclable packaging.
- DIY Solutions: Create DIY solutions for cleaning and personal care to decrease packaging waste and regulate ingredient quality.

2.3. Sustainable Eating

Plant-Based Diet:

- Plant-Rich Meals: Incorporate more plant-based foods into your diet to lower your carbon footprint and boost health.
- Seasonal and Local: Eat seasonal and locally grown produce to promote sustainable agriculture and decrease transportation emissions.

Mindful Eating:

- Food Waste Reduction: Plan meals, store food carefully, and use leftovers creatively to limit food waste.
- Organic Choices: Choose organic foods to avoid pesticides and promote ecologically friendly agricultural techniques.

2.4. Energy Conservation

Energy Efficiency:

- Efficient Appliances: Use energy-efficient appliances and light bulbs to decrease energy usage.
- Renewable Energy: Consider installing solar panels or adopting renewable energy sources for your house.

Everyday Habits:

- Unplug gadgets: Unplug electronic gadgets when not in use to conserve energy.
- Temperature Control: Optimize heating and cooling by utilizing programmable thermostats and weatherproofing your home.

3. The Impact of Sustainable Living on Health and the Environment

3.1. Health Benefits

Physical Health:

- Cleaner Air: Reduced pollution leads to greater respiratory health and lower risk of chronic illnesses.
- Nutritious Diet: Access to organic and locally farmed foods boosts nutrition and maintains energy levels.

Mental and Emotional Well-being:

- Connection to Nature: Sustainable living develops a stronger connection to nature, boosting relaxation and lowering stress.
- Feeling of Purpose: Engaging in eco-friendly behaviors instills a feeling of purpose and responsibility, promoting mental and emotional wellness.

3.2. Environmental Benefits

Resource Conservation:

- Water and Energy Savings: Sustainable methods preserve water and energy, ensuring these resources are accessible for future generations.
- Biodiversity Protection: Supporting sustainable agriculture and decreasing pollution helps conserve biodiversity and ecosystems.

Pollution Reduction:

- Lower Emissions: Reducing waste and energy usage minimizes greenhouse gas emissions, reducing climate change.

- Cleaner Ecosystems: Minimizing chemical usage and waste leads to cleaner soil, water, and air, benefiting all living organisms.

4. Integrating Sustainable Practices into Daily Life

4.1. Setting Goals

Personal Sustainability Goals:

- Specific Objectives: Set precise, measurable targets for adopting eco-friendly behaviors (e.g., "Reduce plastic use by 50% within six months").
- Action Plan: Develop a clear action plan detailing measures to meet your sustainability goals.

4.2. Educating and Engaging Others

Community Involvement:

- Awareness initiatives: Participate in or organize community awareness initiatives to promote sustainable living.
- Collaborative Efforts: Engage with local groups, schools, and companies to promote and execute sustainability programs.

4.3. Continuous Improvement

Ongoing Evaluation:

- Progress Monitoring: Regularly analyze your progress towards sustainability targets and change your tactics as appropriate.
- Learning and Adapting: Stay educated about new sustainable practices and technology, and be open to adapting and enhancing your approach.

Adopting eco-friendly behaviors is a critical component of sustainable living for long-term vitality. By incorporating sustainable consumption, waste reduction, mindful eating, and energy conservation into your everyday life, you may greatly boost your health and well-being while contributing to the health of the world. The benefits of sustainable living extend beyond human health, producing a cleaner, healthier environment for future generations. Embrace sustainable living as a comprehensive approach to vitality, fostering a balanced, aware, and eco-conscious existence.

The Connection between Environment and Well-being

The environment plays a key influence in developing our general well-being. From the air we breathe to the food we consume, our surroundings profoundly affect our physical health, mental mood, and emotional balance. Understanding the significant relationship between the environment and well-being may encourage us to embrace sustainable practices and support healthier lifestyles. This section addresses how diverse environmental issues impact well-being and the efforts we can take to build a better, more sustainable world.

1. Physical Health and the Environment

1.1. Air Quality

Impact on Respiratory Health:

- Pollution: Exposure to pollutants such as particulate matter, nitrogen dioxide, and sulfur dioxide can contribute to respiratory difficulties, including asthma, bronchitis, and other chronic respiratory disorders.
- Clean Air: Access to clean air lessens the risk of respiratory disorders and promotes general lung function, contributing to greater physical health.

1.2. Water Quality

Hydration and Nutrition:

- Polluted Water: Drinking polluted water can lead to different health concerns, including gastrointestinal ailments, neurological disorders, and reproductive troubles.
- Clean Water: Ensuring access to clean, safe drinking water helps hydration, nutrition absorption, and general biological functioning.

1.3. Food Quality

Nutrient Intake:

- Pesticides and Additives: Consuming foods polluted with pesticides, hormones, and artificial additives can affect health, potentially leading to chronic illnesses such as cancer and diabetes.
- Organic and Local Produce: Eating organic, locally sourced foods offers a higher intake of important nutrients while decreasing exposure to hazardous chemicals.

2. Mental Health and the Environment

2.1. Nature and Mental Well-being

Stress Reduction:

- Nature Exposure: Spending time in natural environments, such as parks, woods, and gardens, has been found to reduce stress levels, lower blood pressure, and promote relaxation.
- Green Spaces: Access to green spaces in urban areas gives chances for recreation and relaxation, boosting mental well-being.

2.2. Urbanization and Mental Health

Challenges of Urban Living:

- Noise Pollution: Constant exposure to noise pollution can contribute to increased stress, anxiety, and sleep difficulties.
- Overcrowding: High population density and overcrowding can lead to feelings of isolation, tension, and mental tiredness.

Solutions:

- Urban design: Implementing sensible urban design that incorporates green spaces, noise reduction measures, and communal places can offset these negative impacts and enhance mental health.

3. Emotional Health and the Environment

3.1. Environmental Stressors

Impact of Pollution:

- Chemical Exposure: Exposure to hazardous chemicals and pollutants can disrupt neurological and hormonal systems, leading to emotional disturbances such as mood swings, anxiety, and sadness.
- Environmental Degradation: Living in degraded settings with litter, pollution, and neglected places can lead to feelings of powerlessness and lower emotional well-being.

3.2. Connection to Nature

Emotional Resilience:

- Ecotherapy: Engaging in ecotherapy, which incorporates therapeutic activities in nature, can promote emotional resilience, lessen symptoms of depression, and improve overall emotional health.

- Mindfulness in Nature: Practicing mindfulness and meditation in natural settings builds a deeper connection to the environment and enhances emotional balance and well-being.

4. Creating a Healthy Environment

4.1. Sustainable Practices

Eco-friendly Choices:

Reduce, Reuse, and Recycle: Adopting the concepts of decreasing waste, reusing items, and recycling helps reduce environmental effects and create a healthier living environment.

Sustainable goods: Choosing eco-friendly goods for personal care, cleaning, and home use decreases exposure to dangerous chemicals and encourages a sustainable lifestyle.

4.2. Community Involvement

Collective Action:

- Local efforts: Participating in local environmental efforts, such as community gardens, clean-up drives, and sustainability programs, develops a feeling of community and collective well-being.

- Advocacy and Education: Educating others about the importance of environmental health and pushing for legislation that protects the environment can lead to larger social benefits.

4.3. Personal Habits

Healthy Lifestyle Choices:

- Physical Activity: Incorporating frequent physical activity, especially in natural surroundings, boosts physical and mental health.
- Balanced Diet: Consuming a balanced diet rich in organic, whole foods enhances general well-being and lowers the environmental effect of food production.

The relationship between the environment and well-being is extensive and diverse. A healthy environment improves physical health by providing clean air, water, and nutritional food. It enhances mental well-being through access to green places and less exposure to urban pressures. Emotional health benefits from a clean, natural environment that develops resilience and emotional equilibrium. By adopting sustainable behaviors, participating in community activities, and making thoughtful lifestyle choices, we may increase our well-being and contribute to a healthier, more sustainable world. Embracing the interconnectivity of our environment and well-being allows us to live healthier, more satisfying lives while safeguarding the earth for future generations.

Strategies for a Sustainable and Vital Lifestyle

Adopting a sustainable and vital lifestyle requires making conscious decisions that enhance long-term health and well-being while reducing environmental damage. By integrating eco-friendly habits into everyday routines, individuals can boost their physical health, mental clarity, and emotional balance. This section covers practical ways to establish a sustainable and vital lifestyle, concentrating on aspects such as diet, physical exercise, mental well-being, and community participation.

1. Sustainable Nutrition

1.1. Plant-Based Diet

Benefits:

- Nutrient-Rich: Plant-based diets are rich in important vitamins, minerals, and antioxidants, promoting general health.

- Environmental Impact: Reducing meat consumption minimizes greenhouse gas emissions and conserves water and land resources.

Implementation:

- Gradual Transition: Start by introducing more fruits, veggies, legumes, nuts, and seeds into your meals.
- Meat Alternatives: Explore plant-based proteins such as tofu, tempeh, lentils, and chickpeas to substitute animal products.

1.2. Local and Organic Foods

Benefits:

- Reduced Pesticides: Organic foods are cultivated without synthetic pesticides and fertilizers, encouraging greater health.
- Support for Local Farmers: Buying local produce promotes the local economy and decreases the carbon impact from transportation.

Implementation:

- Farmers' Markets: Shop at farmers' markets to get fresh, local, and organic products.

- Community Supported Agriculture (CSA): Join a CSA program to get regular deliveries of local, seasonal produce.

1.3. Reducing Food Waste

Benefits:

- Resource Conservation: Reducing food waste conserves resources utilized in food production, such as water, energy, and labor.
- Cost Savings: Minimizing waste may cut shopping expenditures and make the most of your food budget.

Implementation:

- Meal Planning: Plan meals ahead of time to buy only what you need and use leftovers creatively.
- Proper Storage: Store food appropriately to increase its shelf life and prevent spoiling.

2. Sustainable Physical Activity

2.1. Outdoor Exercise

Benefits:

- Connection to Nature: Exercising outside increases mental well-being and creates a connection to the environment.

- Variety of Activities: Outdoor activities such as hiking, cycling, and jogging offer various and entertaining ways to keep active.

Implementation:

- Local Trails and Parks: Explore local trails, parks, and nature reserves for frequent outdoor exercise.
- Eco-friendly Gear: Use eco-friendly and sustainable fitness gear manufactured from recycled or natural materials.

2.2. Energy-efficient Workouts

Benefits:

- Reduced Energy Use: Choosing workouts that demand minimum energy use aids sustainability.
- Cost-effective: Low-energy workouts are frequently cost-effective and may be done at home or outdoors.

Implementation:

- Bodyweight Exercises: Practice bodyweight exercises such as push-ups, squats, and yoga that do not require equipment.
- Cycling and Walking: Incorporate cycling and walking into your daily routine as alternatives to driving.

3. Mental and Emotional Well-being

3.1. Mindfulness and Meditation

Benefits:

- Stress Reduction: Mindfulness and meditation activities relieve stress and enhance emotional equilibrium.
- Mental Clarity: Regular meditation promotes attention, clarity, and cognitive function.

Implementation:

- Daily Practice: Set aside time each day for mindfulness or meditation, starting with a few minutes and progressively increasing the duration.
- Nature Meditation: Practice meditation in natural settings to improve your connection to the environment.

3.2. Eco-therapy

Benefits:

- Connection to Nature: Eco-therapy includes connecting with nature to promote mental health and emotional well-being.

- Physical Activity: Many eco-therapy activities, such as gardening or wandering in nature, also give physical health advantages.

Implementation:

- Gardening: Start a garden to grow your veggies, herbs, and flowers, connecting with nature and lowering stress.
- Nature Walks: Regularly take walks in natural environments, such as parks, woods, or beaches.

4. Community and Social Engagement

4.1. Building a Sustainable Community

Benefits:

- Shared Resources: Community initiatives can lead to shared resources and joint action towards sustainability.
- Social Support: Engaging with like-minded folks gives social support and develops sustainable behaviors.

Implementation:

- Community Projects: Participate in or organize community projects focusing on sustainability, such as clean-up drives or tree planting.

- Local Groups: Join local sustainability groups or clubs to network with others and share ideas.

4.2. Educating and Advocating

Benefits:

- Awareness: Educating people about sustainability improves awareness and drives action.
- Policy Change: Advocacy activities can lead to policy changes that favor environmental preservation and sustainability.

Implementation:

- Workshops and Seminars: Attend or host workshops and seminars on sustainability subjects to learn and exchange expertise.
- Advocacy Campaigns: Participate in advocacy campaigns to support sustainable policies and practices at local, regional, and national levels.

Adopting a sustainable and vital lifestyle involves a comprehensive strategy that incorporates diet, physical exercise, mental well-being, and community participation. By adopting thoughtful decisions and integrating eco-friendly activities into everyday routines, individuals may increase their health and vitality while contributing to a more sustainable world. Embracing these tactics produces a balanced, aware, and eco-conscious lifestyle that improves both personal well-being and the environment.

Chapter 12

MAINTAINING ENERGY AND VITALITY AS YOU AGE

Understanding the Aging Process

As we age, our bodies and minds endure many changes that might affect energy levels and vitality. Understanding the aging process is vital for adopting practices that promote health, well-being, and a vigorous existence in later years. This chapter addresses the scientific and psychological elements of aging, the frequent obstacles faced, and how to retain energy and vitality via proactive lifestyle choices.

1. Biological Changes in Aging

1.1. Cellular Aging

Telomere Shortening:

Telomeres are protective caps on the ends of chromosomes that shorten with each cell division, eventually contributing to cellular aging.

Impact:

Shortened telomeres are related to impaired cell function, increased risk of chronic illnesses, and symptoms of aging.

Mitochondrial Function:

- Role: Mitochondria are the powerhouses of cells, providing energy vital for cellular operations.
- Age-related Decline: Mitochondrial efficiency diminishes with age, leading to diminished energy generation and increasing weariness.

1.2. Hormonal Changes

Hormone Levels:

- Estrogen and Testosterone: Levels of sex hormones such as estrogen and testosterone fall with age, influencing energy, muscular mass, and bone density.
- Growth Hormone and DHEA: These hormones also decline, influencing muscle upkeep, skin elasticity, and general vigor.

Impact on Energy:

- Metabolism: Hormonal changes can reduce metabolism, resulting in weight gain and decreased energy.
- Mood and Cognition: Fluctuating hormone levels can alter mood, cognitive performance, and emotional well-being.

1.3. Physical Changes

Muscle Mass and Strength:

- Sarcopenia: Age-related loss of muscle mass and strength, known as sarcopenia, can limit mobility and energy.
- Bone Density: Reduced bone density raises the risk of fractures and osteoporosis, decreasing overall vitality.

Skin and Connective Tissues:

- Elasticity and Hydration: Skin loses elasticity and hydration with age, contributing to wrinkles and dryness.
- Joint Health: Degeneration of cartilage and connective tissues can contribute to joint discomfort and stiffness.

2. Psychological Aspects of Aging

2.1. Cognitive Changes

Memory and Processing Speed:

- Decline: Age-related cognitive decline can decrease memory, processing speed, and problem-solving ability.
- Neuroplasticity: Despite cognitive loss, the brain retains some potential for neuroplasticity, allowing for continuous learning and adaptation.

Mental Health:

- Depression and Anxiety: Older individuals may experience depression and anxiety due to life changes, health challenges, or the death of loved ones.
- Cognitive Health: Maintaining cognitive health is vital for general well-being and quality of life.

2.2. Emotional Changes

Emotional Regulation:

- Increased Resilience: Many older persons gain higher emotional resilience and better coping methods.
- Social Support: Strong social ties and support networks are crucial for emotional health and vitality.

Purpose and Fulfillment:

- Feeling of Purpose: Finding a feeling of purpose and engaging in meaningful activities can boost emotional well-being.
- Lifelong Learning: Continuing to study and explore new interests can bring mental stimulation and happiness.

3. Common Challenges in Aging

3.1. Chronic Health Conditions

Prevalence:

- Common Conditions: Chronic illnesses such as heart disease, diabetes, arthritis, and hypertension grow increasingly frequent with age.
- Treatment: Effective treatment of chronic illnesses is critical for sustaining energy and vigor.

3.2. Mobility and Independence

Mobility concerns:

- Reduced Mobility: Physical limits and mobility concerns can influence independence and quality of life.
- Adaptive techniques: Adopting adaptive techniques and assistive devices can help retain independence.

3.3. Social Isolation

Risks:

- Isolation: Older persons are at risk of social isolation due to retirement, loss of loved ones, or physical restrictions.
- Impact on Health: Social isolation can lead to loneliness, depression, and diminished mental and physical health.

4. Strategies for Maintaining Energy and Vitality

4.1. Healthy Nutrition

Balanced Diet:

- Nutrient-dense Foods: Focus on a diet rich in fruits, vegetables, whole grains, lean meats, and healthy fats.
- Hydration: Stay well-hydrated to maintain overall health and energy levels.

Supplements:

- Vital Nutrients: Consider supplements for vital nutrients such as vitamin D, calcium, and omega-3 fatty acids, after checking with a healthcare practitioner.

4.2. Regular Physical Activity

Exercise Routine:

- Strength Training: Incorporate strength training activities to maintain muscle mass and bone density.
- Aerobic Exercise: Engage in regular aerobic exercises like walking, swimming, or cycling to increase cardiovascular health and energy.

Flexibility and Balance:

- Stretching and Yoga: Practice stretching and yoga to promote flexibility, balance, and joint health.
- Tai Chi: Consider Tai Chi for its gentle motions that enhance balance and minimize fall risk.

4.3. Mental and Emotional Well-being

Cognitive Stimulation:

- Brain Exercises: Engage in activities that engage the brain, such as puzzles, reading, and acquiring new skills.
- Social Engagement: Maintain social relationships through clubs, volunteer work, or community activities.

Emotional Support:

- Therapy and Counseling: Seek therapy or counseling to address emotional difficulties and boost mental health.
- Mindfulness and Relaxation: Practice mindfulness, meditation, and relaxation techniques to manage stress and increase emotional well-being.

4.4. Preventive Healthcare

Regular Check-ups:

- Screenings and Exams: Schedule frequent health check-ups, screenings, and preventative examinations to discover and control health concerns early.
- Vaccinations: Stay up-to-date with vaccines to avoid diseases and maintain health.

Chronic Condition Management:

- Medication Adherence: Follow recommended medication regimes and check chronic conditions regularly.
- Healthy Lifestyle: Adopt a healthy lifestyle to complement medical treatments and enhance outcomes.

Understanding the aging process is critical for retaining energy and vigor as you age. By acknowledging the biological, psychological, and emotional changes that occur with aging, you may adopt proactive methods to promote your health and well-being. A balanced diet, frequent physical exercise, cognitive stimulation, and social involvement are crucial components of a vigorous and meaningful existence in senior years. Embrace these tactics to boost your energy, vitality, and general quality of life, supporting a healthy and active aging process.

Adapting Habits for Lifelong Vitality

Maintaining vitality throughout life includes adopting and adjusting behaviors that enhance physical health, mental well-being, and emotional resiliency. As we age, our bodies and brains change, prompting adaptations to our habits and lifestyles to continue feeling energetic and bright. This section provides fundamental techniques for modifying behaviors to sustain lifetime vitality, concentrating on diet, physical exercise, mental health, and social relationships.

1. Nutrition for Lifelong Vitality

1.1. Embracing a Balanced Diet

Nutrient-Dense Foods:

- Entire Foods: Prioritize entire foods such as fruits, vegetables, whole grains, lean meats, and healthy fats to provide a balanced intake of important nutrients.
- Antioxidant-Rich Foods: Incorporate foods strong in antioxidants, such as berries, leafy greens, and nuts, to battle oxidative stress and maintain cellular health.

Portion Control:

- Mindful Eating: Practice mindful eating by paying attention to hunger and fullness cues, and avoiding overeating.
- Smaller, Frequent Meals: Opt for smaller, more frequent meals to maintain steady energy levels throughout the day.

1.2. Hydration

Importance of Hydration:

- Water Intake: Aim to drink at least eight glasses of water daily to assist digestion, metabolism, and general bodily processes.
- Hydrating Food: Include hydrating foods such as cucumbers, melons, and oranges in your diet to enhance water consumption.

1.3. Adapting to Changing Nutritional Needs

Age-Related Nutritional Adjustments:

- Calcium and Vitamin D: Ensure appropriate intake of calcium and vitamin D to promote bone health, especially when bone density diminishes with age.
- Protein: Increase protein consumption to maintain muscle mass and heal tissues, particularly through lean sources like fish, poultry, and lentils.

2. Physical Activity for Lifelong Vitality

2.1. Regular Exercise Routine

Diverse Activities:

- Aerobic Exercise: Engage in aerobic exercises such as walking, swimming, or cycling to enhance cardiovascular health and endurance.
- Strength Training: Incorporate strength training activities to increase and maintain muscle mass and bone density.

Flexibility and Balance:

- Stretching: Regular stretching exercises assist preserve flexibility, minimize the chance of injury, and enhance general mobility.
- Balance activities: Practice balance activities such as yoga or Tai Chi to strengthen stability and prevent falls.

2.2. Adapting Exercise to Physical Change

Listening to Your Body:

- Modify Intensity: Adjust the intensity and length of workouts based on your fitness level and any physical restrictions.

- Incorporate Rest: Allow ample rest and recovery time to minimize overexertion and assist muscle recovery.

Low-Impact Options:

- Gentle Activities: Opt for low-impact activities like swimming or water aerobics, which are easy on the joints while still delivering decent exercise.
- Adaptive Equipment: Use adaptive equipment, such as resistance bands or adjusted weights, to accommodate physical changes and guarantee safe workout habits.

3. Mental and Emotional Well-being for Lifelong Vitality

3.1. Cognitive Health

Stimulating the Mind:

- Lifetime Learning: Engage in lifetime learning through reading, puzzles, classes, and new interests to keep your mind sharp.
- Mental activities: Practice mental activities like Sudoku, crosswords, and memory games to increase cognitive function.

3.2. Emotional Resilience

Managing Stress:

- Mindfulness and Meditation: Incorporate mindfulness techniques and meditation into your daily routine to decrease stress and create emotional equilibrium.
- Stress-Reduction Techniques: Use strategies such as deep breathing, gradual muscle relaxation, and visualization to handle stress successfully.

3.3. Seeking Support

Professional Help:

- Therapy and Counseling: Seek therapy or counseling to address emotional difficulties, manage stress, and enhance mental health.
- Support Groups: Join support groups to connect with individuals who have similar experiences and give mutual support.

4. Social Connections for Lifelong Vitality

4.1. Building and Maintaining Relationships

Staying Connected:

- Frequent Interaction: Maintain frequent touch with family, friends, and community members through calls, visits, and social activities.

- Community Involvement: Participate in community activities, groups, and volunteer work to be socially active and involved.

4.2. Creating a Supportive Network

Mutual Support:

- Social Support Networks: Build a network of supportive connections that give emotional, practical, and social support.

- Intergenerational Connections: Foster intergenerational relationships by interacting with people of different ages for unique viewpoints and mutual learning.

5. Personal Growth and Adaptation

5.1. Embracing Change

Adaptability:

- Flexibility: Be open to modifying habits and routines to accommodate changes in physical, mental, and emotional health.
- Positive Attitude: Cultivate a positive attitude towards aging, viewing it as a chance for growth and new experiences.

5.2. Setting Realistic Goals

Achievable Milestones:

- Short-term and Long-term objectives: Set reasonable and achievable short-term and long-term objectives for health, fitness, and personal growth.
- Tracking Progress: Regularly measure progress and celebrate milestones to keep inspired and dedicated to your vitality journey.

Adapting behaviors for lifetime vitality entails making intentional modifications to nutrition, physical exercise, mental well-being, and social relationships. By recognizing and adapting to the changes that come with age, you may retain a lively, active, and satisfying life. Embrace the path of lifetime vitality by adopting sustainable behaviors, remaining connected, and always pursuing personal growth and adaptability.

Tips for Staying Active and Engaged in Later Years

Staying active and involved in older years is vital for sustaining physical health, mental sharpness, and emotional well-being. Adopting measures that encourage regular physical exercise, social engagement, and constant learning can increase the quality of life and build a feeling of purpose. This section contains practical advice for keeping active and involved, concentrating on fitness, cerebral stimulation, social participation, and personal growth.

1. Prioritizing Physical Activity

1.1. Regular Exercise Routine

Find Enjoyable Activities:

- Personal Preferences: Choose physical activities that you like, such as walking, swimming, dancing, or gardening, to keep motivated.
- Variety: Incorporate a variety of exercises to train different muscle groups and keep workouts interesting.

Structured Exercise Programs:

- Fitness programs: Join fitness programs geared to elders, such as yoga, Tai Chi, or water aerobics, to keep active in a social atmosphere.

- Personal Trainer: Consider working with a personal trainer who specializes in senior fitness to design a tailored training regimen.

1.2. Staying Active at Home

Home Workouts:

- Online Resources: Utilize online workout videos or fitness applications developed for seniors to exercise at home.

- Simple Equipment: Use basic equipment like resistance bands, small weights, or a chair for support to boost home exercises.

Everyday Movement:

- Household Activities: Incorporate physical exercise into everyday duties like cleaning, gardening, or organizing to keep active throughout the day.

- Walking Breaks: Take regular walking breaks to stretch and exercise, especially if you spend a lot of time sitting.

1.3. Safe and Adaptable Exercises

Low-Impact Activities:

- Gentle on Joints: Engage in low-impact activities like swimming, cycling, or elliptical training to preserve your joints while being active.
- Flexibility Exercises: Incorporate stretching and flexibility exercises to maintain range of motion and lessen the chance of injury.

Adaptive Fitness:

- Mobility Aids: Use mobility aids like walkers or canes if needed, and pick workouts that accommodate any physical restrictions.
- Sat Exercises: Try sat exercises or chair yoga if standing for lengthy periods is problematic.

2. Enhancing Mental Stimulation

2.1. Lifelong Learning

New talents and Hobbies:

- Classes and Workshops: Enroll in classes or workshops to acquire new talents, such as painting, cooking, or a musical instrument.

- Online classes: Explore online classes on sites like Coursera, edX, or Udemy to study new subjects from home.

Creative Activities:

- Art and Crafts: Engage in creative activities like sketching, crocheting, or woodworking to stimulate the mind and express creativity.
- Writing and Journaling: Start a diary, write stories, or create poetry to keep the mind busy and chronicle events.

2.2. Cognitive Exercises

Brain Games:

- Puzzles and Games: Solve puzzles, crosswords, Sudoku, or play card and board games to engage the brain and increase cognitive performance.
- Memory Exercises: Practice memory exercises or tasks that involve recollection and focus to keep the mind sharp.

Reading and Writing:

- Books and Articles: Read books, newspapers, or articles on diverse themes to keep informed and stimulate the mind.
- Discussion Groups: Join book clubs or discussion groups to exchange thoughts and engage in intellectual debates.

3. Fostering Social Connections

3.1. Building Relationships

Family and Friends:

- Regular Visits: Schedule regular visits or calls with family and friends to preserve strong social relationships.
- Family Activities: Participate in family events and gatherings to stay connected and involved.

Community Involvement:

- Volunteer Work: Volunteer for local groups, charities, or community initiatives to give back and meet new people.
- Social Clubs: Join social clubs, senior centers, or hobby organizations that correspond with your interests to make new friends and stay active.

3.2. Embracing Technology

Staying Connected:

- Social Media: Use social media platforms like Facebook, Instagram, or WhatsApp to remain in contact with loved ones and join online groups.
- Video Calls: Utilize video call services like Zoom, Skype, or FaceTime for virtual face-to-face encounters.

Learning and Entertainment:

- Online Communities: Participate in online forums or groups about your hobbies to interact with like-minded folks.

- Digital Entertainment: Explore digital entertainment choices including streaming movies, listening to podcasts, or attending virtual events.

4. Promoting Personal Development

4.1. Setting Goals

Personal Milestones:

- Short-term objectives: Set short-term objectives for exercise, learning, or personal tasks to keep motivated and focused.

- Long-term objectives: Identify long-term objectives and build a strategy to accomplish them, such as traveling, publishing a book, or mastering a new skill.

4.2. Reflecting and Adapting

Self-reflection:

- Journaling: Keep a journal to reflect on your experiences, ideas, and feelings, and monitor progress towards your objectives.
- Mindfulness: Practice mindfulness and meditation to stay present and create a good outlook.

Flexibility and Adaptation:

- Altering Plans: Be open to altering plans and objectives as required based on your physical and mental health.
- Embracing Change: Embrace change and new possibilities with a positive attitude, seeing them as potential for growth and development.

5. Seeking Professional Support

5.1. Medical and Health Services

Frequent Check-ups:

- Preventative Care: Schedule frequent medical check-ups, screenings, and preventative care to monitor and maintain health.

- Specialist Consultations: Consult professionals for any specific health issues or illnesses to obtain tailored care.

5.2. Mental Health Services

Counseling and Therapy:

- Professional Help: Seek counseling or therapy for emotional support, stress management, and mental health maintenance.
- Support Groups: Join support groups for those having similar issues or experiences to share and get assistance.

Staying active and involved in older years is crucial for sustaining physical health, mental clarity, and emotional well-being. By prioritizing regular physical exercise, improving cerebral stimulation, cultivating social relationships, stimulating personal growth, and obtaining professional help, you may enjoy a meaningful and vibrant life.

Chapter 13

REAL-LIFE SUCCESS STORIES

Inspiring Case Studies

Reading about real-life success stories can be incredibly motivating and provide tangible examples of how adopting healthy habits and making positive lifestyle changes can lead to remarkable improvements in energy and vitality. This chapter showcases inspiring case studies of individuals who have transformed their lives by embracing wellness principles. Their journeys highlight the power of commitment, resilience, and the impact of healthy choices on overall well-being.

Case Study 1: John's Journey to Renewed Vitality

Background:

John, a retired school teacher in his late 60s, struggled with low energy levels, chronic pain, and feelings of isolation after losing his spouse. He realized that his sedentary lifestyle and poor eating habits were contributing to his declining health and decided to make a change.

Approach:

- Physical Activity: John started with gentle exercises, such as walking and chair yoga, gradually increasing the intensity as his fitness improved. He joined a local senior fitness class, which provided both exercise and social interaction.

- Nutrition: He consulted a nutritionist and revamped his diet, focusing on whole foods, lean proteins, and plenty of fruits and vegetables. He also ensured he stayed hydrated throughout the day.

- Social Engagement: To combat loneliness, John joined a community center and participated in volunteer activities, which helped him build new friendships and stay engaged.

Results:

Within six months, John experienced a significant improvement in his energy levels and overall mood. His chronic pain reduced, and he felt more connected and purposeful. John's story exemplifies how a balanced approach to physical activity, nutrition, and social engagement can transform one's health and vitality.

Case Study 2: Maria's Transformation through Holistic Health

Background:

Maria, a 55-year-old business executive, faced burnout from long working hours and high stress. She suffered from poor sleep, weight gain, and frequent headaches. Realizing the need for a holistic approach to health, Maria sought ways to regain her vitality.

Approach:

- Mindfulness and Meditation: Maria incorporated daily mindfulness practices and meditation into her routine to manage stress and improve mental clarity.
- Exercise: She started a fitness regimen that included both cardiovascular exercises and strength training, as well as weekly yoga sessions to enhance flexibility and relaxation.
- Diet and Hydration: Maria adopted a balanced diet rich in superfoods and focused on staying well-hydrated. She also practiced mindful eating to avoid overeating and improve digestion.

Results:

Maria's holistic approach led to a remarkable transformation. She lost weight, improved her sleep quality, and felt more energetic and focused at work. Her headaches diminished, and she experienced a greater sense of well-being. Maria's story highlights the effectiveness of integrating mindfulness, exercise, and proper nutrition for achieving holistic health.

Case Study 3: David's Recovery and Resilience

Background:

David, a 70-year-old retired engineer, suffered a major setback when he was diagnosed with type 2 diabetes. He felt overwhelmed and fearful about his future health. Determined to take control of his condition, David embarked on a journey to improve his lifestyle.

Approach:

- Physical Activity: David began with simple daily walks and gradually incorporated more vigorous activities like swimming and cycling. He worked with a fitness coach to develop a safe and effective exercise plan.
- Nutrition: He followed a diet plan designed to manage his diabetes, focusing on low-glycemic foods, whole grains, and plenty of vegetables. He also monitored his blood sugar levels regularly.
- Education and Support: David educated himself about diabetes management and joined a support group for

individuals with diabetes, which provided encouragement and shared experiences.

Results:

David successfully managed his diabetes, reducing his medication needs and achieving stable blood sugar levels. He lost weight, gained strength, and felt more empowered and resilient. His journey illustrates the importance of education, support, and proactive lifestyle changes in managing chronic conditions and enhancing vitality.

Case Study 4: Linda's Path to Emotional and Physical Wellness

Background:

Linda, a 62-year-old artist, experienced severe anxiety and fatigue following a major life transition. She felt disconnected from her passions and struggled to find joy in daily activities. Seeking a way to reclaim her vitality, Linda embraced a comprehensive wellness plan.

Approach:

- Creative Expression: Linda reignited her passion for art by dedicating time to painting and participating in local art exhibitions. This creative outlet became a source of joy and relaxation.

- Physical Activity: She incorporated regular physical activity, including dance classes and nature hikes, which not only improved her fitness but also lifted her spirits.
- Mental Health: Linda sought therapy to address her anxiety and developed coping strategies to manage stress. She also practiced gratitude journaling and positive affirmations.

Results:

Linda's renewed focus on creative expression, physical activity, and mental health led to a significant improvement in her overall well-being. She felt more energetic, emotionally balanced, and inspired. Linda's story demonstrates the powerful connection between emotional health and physical vitality.

These inspiring case studies highlight the transformative potential of adopting healthy habits and making positive lifestyle changes. Each individual's journey underscores the importance of a holistic approach to wellness, encompassing physical activity, nutrition, mental health, and social engagement. By learning from these real-life success stories, readers can find motivation and practical strategies to enhance their own energy and vitality.

Lessons Learned from the Transformations in Health Situations

Lifestyle changes may have a significant influence on an individual's overall well-being, and health transitions frequently serve as potent reminders of this impact. We can gain useful insights and practical solutions that can be applied to our own lives if we investigate the accomplishments and problems that persons who have achieved major gains in their health have encountered. The purpose of this section is to summarize the most important takeaways from actual health transformations, with a particular emphasis on the significance of dedication, adaptability, holistic methods, and support networks.

1. Commitment to Long-Term Objectives is the First Step

1.1. Establishing Objectives that are both Realistic and Attainable

Gradual Progress:

- Small Step: Instead of attempting to completely revamp your way of life, begin with adjustments that are doable and quite little. Momentum and self-assurance are nurtured by steady advancement.
- More Particular Objectives: To offer clear direction and incentive, it is important to establish SMART goals, which

stands for specified, measurable, attainable, relevant, and time-bound.

1.2. Consistency and Perseverance

Daily Habits:

- Routine Development: Establish routines that combine healthy habits, making them a natural part of your life.
- Consistency Over Perfection: Focus on persistent effort rather than striving for perfection. Small, persistent acts lead to substantial outcomes over time.

2. Adaptability and Flexibility

2.1. Listening to Your Body

Self-Awareness:

- Body Signals: Pay attention to your body's signals and change your actions and habits appropriately. Rest when required and push yourself when you feel competent.
- Health Monitoring: Regularly monitor critical health indicators, such as weight, blood pressure, and blood sugar levels, to evaluate progress and make informed adjustments.

2.2. Embracing Change

Adapting to Circumstances:

- Life Transitions: Be prepared to alter your health habits in response to life changes, such as aging, changing job schedules, or family obligations.
- Flexibility in strategy: Stay open to attempting new ways or tactics if your present strategy isn't providing the intended outcomes.

3. Holistic Health Approaches

3.1. Integrating Multiple Wellness Aspects

Balanced Approach:

- Physical, Mental, and Emotional Health: Recognize that genuine vitality comprises physical fitness, mental clarity, and emotional well-being. Address all components for total health.
- Mind-Body Connection: Practice activities that promote the mind-body connection, such as yoga, meditation, or Tai Chi, to increase overall well-being.

3.2. Sustainable Lifestyle Changes

Long-Term Viability:

- Practical modifications: Implement changes that are sustainable in the long term, avoiding excessive diets or exercise regimens that are difficult to maintain.
- Enjoyable Practices: Choose hobbies and habits that you love and look forward to, making it simpler to continue with them over time.

4. Importance of Support Systems

4.1. Building a Supportive Network

Social Connections:

- Family and Friends: Lean on family and friends for support, accountability, and companionship throughout your health journey.
- Community Involvement: Engage with community groups, exercise programs, or clubs that share your interests and ambitions.

4.2. Professional Guidance

Expert Advice:

- Healthcare Professionals: Consult with healthcare providers, nutritionists, fitness trainers, and mental health counselors to obtain tailored direction and support.
- Educational Resources: Utilize books, online courses, and trusted websites to educate yourself on health and wellness themes.

5. Mindset and Motivation

5.1. Positive Attitude

Optimism:

- Focus on Positives: Maintain a positive attitude towards your health journey, appreciating minor successes and progress rather than obsessing over failures.
- Resilience: Cultivate resilience by viewing obstacles as opportunities to learn and grow.

5.2. Intrinsic Motivation

Internal Drive:

- Personal Reasons: Identify and focus on personal reasons for wanting to improve your health, such as improved energy, better quality of life, or the capacity to engage in activities you enjoy.
- Self-Reflection: Regularly reflect on your success and remind yourself of the rewards you've received from your efforts.

The lessons acquired from health transitions underscore the significance of dedication, adaptation, comprehensive methods, support structures, and a positive outlook. By integrating these principles into your health journey, you may develop a lasting and enjoyable road to enhanced energy and vitality. Embrace the process, be open to learning, and seek help as required to attain permanent health and well-being.

How to Apply These Lessons to Your Own Life

Applying the lessons learned from health transitions to your own life can help you achieve sustained increases in energy, vitality, and general well-being. By integrating practical tactics and a holistic approach, you may design a tailored strategy that corresponds with your particular requirements and goals. Here's how you can successfully utilize these lessons:

1. Commit to Long-Term Goals

1.1. Set Realistic and Achievable Goals

Start Small:

- Initial Steps: Begin with simple, realistic objectives that are easy to include in your everyday routine. For example, start with a 10-minute walk each day or substitute sugary snacks with fruit.
- SMART Goals: Use the SMART criteria (Specific, Measurable, Achievable, Relevant, Time-bound) to develop clear and realistic goals. This can offer direction and a sense of success.

1.2. Build Consistency

Everyday behaviors:

- Routine Integration: Incorporate healthy behaviors into your everyday routine. Consistent activities, no matter how modest, compound over time and lead to big changes.
- Track Progress: Keep a journal or use a tracking tool to record your progress. This helps sustain motivation and delivers a sense of success.

2. Embrace Adaptability and Flexibility

2.1. Listen to Your Body

Self-Awareness:

- Body Signals: Pay heed to your body's cues, such as exhaustion, discomfort, or hunger. Adjust your activity and food accordingly to preserve balance and avoid burnout.
- Regular Check-ins: Schedule regular self-assessments or check-ins with a healthcare practitioner to evaluate your health and make any modifications.

2.2. Be Open to Change

Flexibility:

- Adapt to Circumstances: Be prepared to adapt your routines in response to life changes, such as job schedules, family responsibilities, or health concerns.
- Experiment and Learn: Don't be scared to attempt new techniques or activities. If something isn't working, review and change your plan.

3. Adopt a Holistic Health Approach

3.1. Balance Multiple Wellness Aspects

Comprehensive Care:

- Physical, Mental, Emotional Health: Address all elements of your well-being. Include physical activities, mental exercises, and emotional self-care in your regimen.
- Mind-Body activities: Incorporate activities like yoga, meditation, or Tai Chi to increase the link between mind and body.

3.2. Focus on Sustainability

Long-Term improvements:

- Practical Adjustments: Implement improvements that are sustainable in the long term. Avoid excessive diets or rigorous exercise routines that may be difficult to sustain.
- Enjoyable Activities: Choose activities and dietary adjustments that you enjoy. This raises the probability of continuing with them over time.

4. Build a Supportive Network

4.1. Leverage Social Connections

Community Involvement:

- Family and Friends: Engage your family and friends in your health journey. Their support and friendship can give drive and accountability.
- Join Groups: Participate in community groups, exercise classes, or clubs that coincide with your interests. This encourages social relationships and shared experiences.

4.2. Seek Professional Guidance

Expert assistance:

- Healthcare Professionals: Consult with healthcare experts, nutritionists, fitness trainers, and mental health counselors to obtain tailored guidance and assistance.
- Educational Resources: Utilize books, online courses, and trusted websites to educate yourself on health and wellness themes.

5. Cultivate a Positive Mindset

5.1. Maintain a Positive Attitude

Optimism:

- Focus on Progress: Celebrate minor successes and progress rather than obsessing over failures. A cheerful mindset can boost motivation and resilience.
- Resilience: View obstacles as chances to learn and improve. Cultivate resilience by embracing failures as part of the process.

5.2. Foster Intrinsic Motivation

Internal Drive:

- Personal Reasons: Identify and focus on personal reasons for improving your health, such as improved energy, better quality of life, or the capacity to engage in activities you enjoy.
- Self-Reflection: Regularly reflect on your success and remind yourself of the rewards you've received from your efforts.

Applying the lessons from health changes to your own life entails setting realistic objectives, accepting adaptation, taking a holistic approach, developing a supporting network, and maintaining a positive mentality. By incorporating these tactics, you may establish a sustainable and enjoyable route to greater energy and vitality. Embrace the journey, be open to learning, and seek help as required to attain sustainable health and well-being.

Chapter 14

TOOLS AND RESOURCES FOR CONTINUED GROWTH

Recommended Books, Apps, and Websites

As you embark on your journey toward improved energy and vitality, leveraging various tools and resources can support and enhance your efforts. This chapter provides a curated selection of books, apps, and websites designed to offer valuable information, practical advice, and ongoing motivation. These resources will help you stay informed, track your progress, and continue growing in your pursuit of well-being.

Recommended Books

1. The Glucose Goddess Nutritious Diet Plan: The 4-Week Plan to Curb Cravings, Boost Energy, and Feel Incredible. ***Author:*** Dr. Jessica Reeves

Why Should Read This Book:

- **The Glucose Goddess Nutritious Diet Plan** is ideal for anyone looking to improve their health and wellness through balanced nutrition. Whether you want to manage your weight, boost your energy levels, enhance mental clarity, or simply adopt healthier eating habits, this book provides the tools and knowledge you need to succeed.

2. Glucose Transformation into Diet: The Astonishing Benefits of Maintaining Stable Blood Sugar Levels" by *Dr. Jessica Reeves* is a comprehensive guide that reveals the transformative power of balanced blood sugar for achieving optimal health and well-being. This book explores the critical connection between diet and glucose management, offering readers practical strategies and insights to maintain stable blood sugar levels through dietary adjustments and lifestyle changes.

Why You Should Read This Book:

- **Glucose Transformation into Diet:** The Astonishing Benefits of Maintaining Stable Blood Sugar Levels***"** offers a revolutionary approach to managing your health through balanced blood sugar. Authored by renowned nutritional expert Dr. Jessica Reeves, this guide provides practical strategies, customizable meal plans, and expert insights to help you achieve optimal well-being. Whether you're managing diabetes, pre-diabetes, or simply aiming for better health, this book equips you with the tools to make informed dietary choices, improve energy levels, and enhance overall vitality. Embrace a healthier lifestyle with actionable advice from a trusted authority in nutritional health.

Recommended links

- https://www.amazon.com/dp/B0D934CLVW
- https://www.amazon.com/dp/B0D9PMGT6Y

Scan QR Code

Recommended Apps

1. MyFitnessPal

- Overview: MyFitnessPal is a popular app for tracking diet and exercise, providing detailed insights into your nutritional intake and physical activity.
- Features: Food diary, exercise log, barcode scanner, and integration with other fitness apps.

2. Headspace

- Overview: Headspace offers guided meditation and mindfulness exercises to help manage stress and improve mental clarity.
- Features: Meditation sessions, sleep aids, mindfulness practices, and progress tracking.

3. Fitbit

- Overview: The Fitbit app works with Fitbit devices to monitor physical activity, sleep, and overall health metrics.
- Features: Activity tracking, sleep analysis, heart rate monitoring, and goal setting.

4. Calm

- Overview: Calm provides a range of resources for relaxation, including guided meditations, sleep stories, and breathing exercises.
- Features: Meditation sessions, sleep aids, relaxation music, and daily calm exercises.

5. Yummly

- Overview: Yummly offers personalized recipe recommendations and meal planning features based on your dietary preferences and goals.
- Features: Recipe discovery, meal planning, shopping lists, and nutritional information.

Leveraging books, apps, and links can greatly enhance your journey toward improved energy and vitality. These resources offer valuable information, practical tools, and ongoing support to help you stay informed, track your progress, and continue growing in your pursuit of well-being. By integrating these tools into your routine, you can foster lasting positive changes and achieve your health goals.

Finding Professional Support and Guidance

Navigating the route toward greater energy and vitality may be challenging, and obtaining expert advice and direction can considerably boost your efforts. Professionals such as healthcare specialists, nutritionists, fitness experts, and mental health counselors offer specialized expertise and individualized recommendations that can help you reach your health objectives efficiently. This section covers how to discover and work with several sorts of specialists to help your health journey.

1. Identifying the Right Professionals

1.1. Healthcare Providers

Role:

- General Practitioners (GPs): Offer comprehensive medical treatment, do routine check-ups, and manage chronic illnesses. They can make recommendations to experts if needed.

- Internists and Specialists: Address particular health problems, such as cardiologists for heart health or endocrinologists for diabetes control.

How to Find:

- Referrals: Seek referrals from friends, relatives, or your primary care physician.
- Professional Associations: Use directories from organizations such as the American Medical Association (AMA) or equivalent groups in your country.

1.2. Nutritionists and Dietitians

Role:

- Registered Dietitians (RDs): Provide evidence-based dietary recommendations customized to your particular health requirements and objectives. They can aid with meal planning, managing dietary restrictions, and increasing general nutrition.
- Certified Nutritionists: Offer tailored dietary guidance and help for reaching particular health targets.

How to Find:

- Professional societies: Look for RDs through organizations like the Academy of Nutrition and Dietetics or equivalent local societies.
- Internet Directories: Use Internet directories or health service platforms to identify skilled nutrition providers.

1.3. Fitness Experts

Role:

- Personal Trainers: Design tailored workout plans depending on your fitness level, goals, and any medical issues. They give incentives, instruction, and accountability.
- Exercise Physiologists: Specialize in establishing exercise regimens for patients with chronic health issues or those undergoing rehabilitation.

How to Find:

- Certifying Bodies: Find certified trainers through organizations such as the American Council on Exercise (ACE) or the National Academy of Sports Medicine (NASM).
- Local Gyms & Fitness Centers: Many fitness establishments have qualified trainers on staff who may give personal training sessions.

1.4. Mental Health Counselors

Role:

- Therapists and Psychologists: Provide help for managing stress, anxiety, depression, and other mental health difficulties. They employ numerous therapy strategies to assist promote emotional well-being.

- Licensed Clinical Social Workers (LCSWs): Offer counseling and assistance for emotional and mental health difficulties, frequently with an emphasis on practical solutions and support.

How to Find:

- Professional Associations: Locate mental health specialists through organizations like the American Psychological Association (APA) or comparable institutions.
- Referrals and Reviews: Seek referrals from healthcare practitioners or read reviews on mental health directories.

2. How to Choose the Right Professional

2.1. Assess Qualifications and Experience

Credentials:

- Verify Credentials: Ensure that the expert has adequate credentials, certificates, and licenses related to their specialty.
- Experience: Consider their experience in dealing with difficulties comparable to yours, such as chronic health disorders or specific wellness objectives.

2.2. Evaluate Compatibility and Approach

Personal Fit:

- Communication Style: Choose a professional whose communication style and approach correspond with your preferences. A good rapport can boost the efficacy of your sessions.
- Treatment Philosophy: Ensure their treatment philosophy and procedures correspond with your beliefs and aims.

2.3. Consider Accessibility and Availability

Location and Scheduling:

- Convenience: Choose a professional whose location and hours are convenient for you. Consider possibilities for virtual consultations if in-person meetings are hard.
- Availability: Check their availability and ensure they can meet your schedule for regular appointments.

3. Making the Most of Professional Support

3.1. Set Clear Goals

Objective Setting:

- Define objectives: Establish your health and wellbeing objectives before consulting with a specialist. This lets them personalize their recommendations and solutions to your requirements.

- Discuss Expectations: Communicate your expectations and any issues you may have to ensure a collaborative approach.

3.2. Follow Recommendations and Feedback

Action Plan:

- Implement Advice: Actively follow the advice and action plans offered by your professional. Consistent commitment to their instruction is vital for achieving success.
- Provide input: Share input on what is working and what may require improvement. Open communication enables for continuing development of your plan.

3.3. Track Progress

Monitoring:

- Progress Tracking: Regularly document your progress towards your objectives, utilizing tools or journals as advised by your expert.
- Review Sessions: Schedule frequent evaluations to assess your progress and make required revisions to your plan.

Finding and working with the correct specialists may dramatically assist your journey toward greater energy and vitality. By selecting skilled healthcare doctors, dietitians, fitness experts, and mental health counselors, and by picking specialists whose approach corresponds with your goals, you may obtain individualized assistance and direction. Leveraging professional experience, creating specific goals, and actively engaging in your wellness plan will help you achieve permanent health improvements and maintain vitality.

Building Your Wellness Toolkit

A personal wellness toolbox is a collection of materials, practices, and techniques personalized to promote your health and well-being. This toolbox helps you maintain balance, manage stress, and retain energy and vitality throughout your everyday life. Building a complete wellness toolbox entails combining many parts that address physical, mental, and emotional well-being. Here's how to design and utilize your wellness toolkit efficiently.

1. Assessing Your Needs

1.1. Self-Reflection

Identify Priorities:

- Health objectives: Reflect on your present health state and create your wellness objectives. Consider areas such as physical fitness, diet, sleep, mental health, and stress management.
- Lifestyle Factors: Assess your daily routines, habits, and lifestyle aspects that impact your well-being. Identify areas where you'd like to see progress or change.

1.2. Personalized Approach

Tailored Strategies:

- Individual requirements: Recognize that everyone's wellness requirements are unique. Consider considerations such as age, health issues, interests, and lifestyle while developing your toolset.
- Holistic View: Adopt a holistic approach that addresses all elements of your well-being, including physical, mental, emotional, and social health.

2. Essential Components of a Wellness Toolkit

2.1. Physical Health

Exercise and Movement:

- Activity Plan: Develop a regular exercise regimen that incorporates cardiovascular, strength, flexibility, and balance activities. Tailor the plan to your fitness level and taste.

- Incorporate Movement: Integrate movement into your regular tasks, such as taking short walks, using stairs, or stretching during breaks.

Nutrition:

- Balanced Diet: Create a meal plan that prioritizes healthy foods, balanced macronutrients, and enough water. Include a mix of fruits, vegetables, lean meats, whole grains, and healthy fats.

- Smart Eating Habits: Practice mindful eating, portion management, and regular meal scheduling to ensure sustained energy levels.

2.2. Mental and Emotional Health

Mindfulness and Meditation:

- Mindfulness Practices: Incorporate mindfulness activities such as deep breathing, meditation, and body scans to reduce stress and promote mental clarity.
- Daily Meditation: Set aside time each day for meditation to achieve relaxation and emotional equilibrium.

Stress Management:

- Relaxation Techniques: Use strategies such as progressive muscle relaxation, guided imagery, or aromatherapy to reduce stress and promote relaxation.
- Creative Outlets: Engage in creative hobbies like writing, sketching, or performing music to express feelings and reduce stress.

2.3. Sleep and Rest

Sleep Hygiene:

- Healthy Sleep Habits: Establish a consistent sleep schedule, establish a tranquil sleep environment, and avoid stimulants before bedtime.

- Restorative Practices: Include brief naps, rest breaks, and relaxation activities throughout the day to recharge and prevent burnout.

2.4. Social Connections

Building ties:

- Support Network: Cultivate ties with family, friends, and community people who give emotional support and companionship.
- Social Activities: Participate in social activities, clubs, or groups that correspond with your interests and boost your sense of belonging.

3. Tools and Resources

3.1. Digital Tools

Health and Wellness Apps:

- Fitness Trackers: Use apps like Fitbit, MyFitnessPal, or Apple Health to monitor physical activity, nutrition, and sleep habits.
- Meditation and Mindfulness: Apps such as Headspace, Calm, or Insight Timer provide guided meditation, mindfulness exercises, and relaxation techniques.

Online Resources:

- Educational Websites: Access credible health information, articles, and resources from websites like Healthline, Mayo Clinic, and WebMD.
- Virtual Communities: Join online forums, support groups, or social media communities focusing on health and wellness themes.

3.2. Physical Tools

Exercise Equipment:

- Home Gym Essentials: Invest in basic exercise equipment such as resistance bands, dumbbells, yoga mats, or stability balls for home exercises.
- Wearable Devices: Consider wearable fitness trackers or smartwatches to monitor your activity levels, heart rate, and sleep quality.

Wellness Accessories:

- Relaxation Aids: Use products like essential oil diffusers, weighted blankets, or stress balls to aid relaxation and stress reduction.

- Nutritional Support: Keep a stock of nutritious snacks, meal prep containers, and water bottles to support your dietary objectives.

4. Creating a Routine

4.1. Daily Schedule

Structured Routine:

- Consistent Habits: Establish a daily routine that combines your wellness routines. Consistency helps establish beneficial behaviors and fosters long-term well-being.
- Balanced Activities: Allocate time for physical exercise, relaxation, social connections, and self-care within your daily calendar.

4.2. Flexibility and Adaptability

Change as Needed:

- Listen to Your Body: Be alert to your body's messages and change your routine as required. Flexibility permits you to adjust to changing requirements and circumstances.
- Periodic Reviews: Regularly examine and update your wellness toolbox to ensure it continues to fit your developing objectives and preferences.

5. Seeking Professional Support

5.1. Expert Guidance

Healthcare Providers:

- Regular Check-Ups: Schedule routine medical check-ups and screenings to monitor your health condition and address any issues.
- Professional Advice: Consult with healthcare doctors, nutritionists, fitness experts, and mental health counselors for tailored guidance and support.

5.2. Community Resources

Local Programs:

- Wellness seminars: Participate in community wellness programs, seminars, or classes that give knowledge and support on different health concerns.
- Support Groups: Join local or virtual support groups focusing on specific health conditions or wellness objectives to obtain insights and encouragement from others.

Building your wellness toolbox entails analyzing your requirements, combining critical components of physical, mental, and emotional health, and employing a range of tools and resources. By building a scheduled yet flexible routine, using digital and physical resources, and seeking expert guidance, you may develop a thorough and successful health plan. This toolbox will enable you to maintain balance, control stress, and retain energy and vitality throughout your everyday life, eventually leading to long-term well-being and joy.

Chapter 15

THE JOURNEY AHEAD

Setting Long-term Goals

Setting long-term objectives is a critical element of sustaining continuous energy and vigor. These goals give direction, inspiration, and a clear path for your health journey. Long-term objectives help you keep focused on the wider picture and allow for ongoing progress in your overall well-being. Here's how to properly create and pursue long-term health objectives.

1. Understanding the Importance of Long-term Goals

1.1. Vision and Purpose

Defining Your Vision:

- Clarity: Having a clear vision of what you want to achieve in the long term offers a feeling of purpose and direction. This vision functions as a guiding light, helping you make decisions that match your ultimate health objectives.

- Motivation: Long-term objectives encourage and drive you to continue dedicated to your wellness path, especially when faced with setbacks.

1.2. Continuous Improvement

Ongoing Progress:

- Sustained Efforts: Long-term objectives inspire continual efforts toward progress, developing an attitude of lifelong health and vigor.
- Adaptability: They give a foundation for adjusting and evolving your methods as your requirements and circumstances change over time.

2. Setting Effective Long-term Goals

2.1. SMART Goals

Specific, Measurable, Achievable, Relevant, Time-bound:

- Specific: Clearly state what you intend to achieve. Avoid broad words; instead, define the specific conclusion you intend.
- Measurable: Establish criteria for monitoring development. Quantifiable objectives help you to track your advancements and know when you've reached them.
- Achievable: Set realistic objectives that are feasible given your existing circumstances and resources. Aim for demanding yet realistic aims.

- Relevant: Ensure your goals are connected with your overall vision and personal beliefs. They should be significant to you.
- Time-bound: Assign a timetable to your goals. Having deadlines provides a sense of urgency and helps you stay focused.

Examples:

- Health: "I will reduce my body fat percentage by 5% within the next 12 months through regular exercise and a balanced diet."
- Fitness: "I will run a half-marathon within the next year by following a structured training program."
- Nutrition: "I will incorporate at least five servings of fruits and vegetables into my daily diet over the next six months."

Break Down Goals

Step-by-Step Approach:

- Milestones: Break down long-term goals into smaller, doable milestones. This makes the process less intimidating and allows for regular accomplishments.

- Short-term Objectives: Identify short-term objectives that lead up to your long-term goals. These work as stepping stones, keeping you on track and inspired.

Example:

- Long-term Goal: "I will achieve and maintain a healthy weight within the next year."
- Milestones: "Lose 2 pounds per month," "Incorporate 30 minutes of exercise daily," "Reduce intake of sugary foods."

3. Creating an Action Plan

3.1. Detailed Planning

Action Steps:

- Explain steps: Clearly explain the exact steps you need to take to attain your goals. This comprises daily, weekly, and monthly responsibilities.
- Resources: Identify the resources and help you need, such as instructional materials, professional guidance, or equipment.

3.2. Monitoring and Evaluation

Track Progress:

- Regular Check-ins: Schedule regular check-ins to analyze your progress. Use notebooks, apps, or other tracking tools to document your successes and difficulties.
- Adjustments: Be flexible and willing to change your action plan as needed. If you find barriers, review your strategy and make appropriate modifications.

4. Staying Motivated and Committed

4.1. Accountability

Support Systems:

- Accountability Partners: Engage with friends, family, or wellness coaches who can hold you responsible and give encouragement.
- Community: Join groups or online communities with similar health aims. Sharing experiences and progress can enhance motivation.

4.2. Celebrating Achievements

Recognize Success:

- Milestone Rewards: Celebrate your successes as you hit major milestones. This promotes positive behavior and keeps you motivated.
- Reflect on Progress: Regularly reflect on how far you've come. Acknowledging your progress, no matter how modest helps maintain a positive mindset.

5. Overcoming Challenges

5.1. Resilience and Perseverance

Facing Setbacks:

- Anticipate Challenges: Recognize that setbacks are a normal part of any endeavor. Prepare psychologically to meet problems with resilience.
- Learn from Failures: View obstacles as chances to learn and improve. Analyze what went wrong, adapt your plan, and continue going ahead.

5.2. Seeking Support

Professional help:

- Consult Experts: When experiencing chronic issues, seek help from specialists such as healthcare providers, dietitians, or fitness trainers.
- Emotional help: Don't hesitate to call out for emotional help from friends, family, or mental health counselors.

Setting long-term objectives is an important component of maintaining continuous energy and vigor. By recognizing the importance of these objectives, adopting the SMART framework, establishing comprehensive action plans, and staying motivated and resilient, you may accomplish major gains in your overall well-being. Remember that your wellness journey is a lifelong process of ongoing development and adaptation. Embrace the trip ahead with dedication, and allow your long-term objectives to guide you toward a better, more vibrant existence.

Staying Motivated and Focused

Maintaining motivation and focus is key to accomplishing long-term health and fitness objectives. It's natural to meet roadblocks and moments of low motivation, but with the appropriate techniques, you can stay on track and continue working toward your ambitions. Here's how to build and keep motivation and attention throughout your wellness journey.

1. Understanding Motivation

1.1. Intrinsic vs. Extrinsic Motivation

Intrinsic Motivation:

- Personal Fulfillment: Intrinsic motivation originates from inside and is motivated by personal fulfillment and happiness. Pursuing things that you like and find rewarding can maintain long-term dedication.
- Autonomy and Mastery: Feeling in control of your goals and experiencing ongoing development can promote intrinsic motivation.

Extrinsic Motivation:

- External Rewards: Extrinsic motivation is motivated by external variables such as rewards, recognition, or avoiding negative consequences. While it might jumpstart your path, the intrinsic drive is frequently more lasting.
- Accountability: External accountability, such as commitments to a trainer or a support group, can help promote extrinsic motivation.

1.2. Finding Your "Why"

Purpose and Meaning:

- Clarify Your Goals: Comprehend why you desire to reach your health objectives. Is it to feel more energetic, enhance your quality of life, or be a role model for your family?
- Deep Connection: Connect your aims to your values and beliefs. This personal connection can create a strong motivating basis.

2. Setting Achievable Milestones

2.1. Break Down Goals

Small Steps:

- Short-term Milestones: Break down your long-term goals into smaller, doable milestones. This makes the trip less intimidating and allows for recurring triumphs.
- Progressive Challenges: Gradually raise the complexity and difficulty of your goals to keep pushing yourself without growing frustrated.

2.2. Track and Celebrate Progress

Visual Tracking:

- Progress Logs: Use diaries, apps, or charts to graphically track your progress. Seeing physical proof of your work may enhance motivation.
- Appreciate Successes: Recognize and appreciate each milestone attained. Rewarding oneself helps promote positive behavior and preserve motivation.

3. Creating a Supportive Environment

3.1. Social Support

Engage with Others:

- Accountability Partners: Partner with friends, family, or coworkers who share similar goals. Regular check-ins can bring reciprocal encouragement and accountability.
- Support Groups: Join support groups or communities focusing on health and wellbeing. Sharing experiences and suggestions can create inspiration and lessen feelings of loneliness.

3.2. Optimize Your Environment

Remove Barriers:

- Healthy Habits: Create an atmosphere that supports your goals. For example, equip your kitchen with nutritious foods, set up a separate workout room, or establish a peaceful sleep environment.
- Minimize Distractions: Identify and minimize distractions that might divert your attention. Create a regimen and keep to it as regularly as possible.

4. Developing Mental Resilience

4.1. Positive Mindset

Growth Mindset:

- Embrace Challenges: View obstacles and disappointments as chances to learn and improve. A growth mentality emphasizes tenacity and resilience.
- Self-Compassion: Practice self-compassion and avoid harsh self-criticism. Acknowledge your efforts and development, even if they are not flawless.

4.2. Stress Management

Relaxation Techniques:

- Mindfulness and Meditation: Incorporate mindfulness techniques and meditation into your everyday routine to decrease stress and boost focus.
- Stress Relievers: Identify stress-relief activities that work for you, such as deep breathing exercises, yoga, or indulging in hobbies.

5. Staying Flexible and Adaptable

5.1. Regular Reassessment

Evaluate and Adjust:

- Periodic Reviews: Regularly examine your objectives, methods, and progress. Adjust your action plan as required to keep aligned with your developing requirements and circumstances.
- Feedback Loop: Use feedback from your progress monitoring to make educated improvements. Flexibility permits you to overcome obstacles and sustain momentum.

5.2. Embrace Change

Alter to Life's Changes:

- Life Transitions: Be prepared to alter your objectives and tactics throughout big life changes, such as a new job, moving, or health concerns.
- Be dedicated: Even when alterations are necessary, be dedicated to your broader vision and long-term objectives.

Staying motivated and focused on your health path involves a combination of inner and extrinsic drive, clear goal-setting, a supportive environment, mental resilience, and adaptability. By recognizing your fundamental motivations, setting manageable milestones, forming a supporting network, having a positive mentality, and being adaptable, you can sustain the desire and focus needed to reach your long-term health objectives. Remember that the path is continuous, and keeping motivation is an ongoing process that changes with you.

Embracing the Continuous Journey of Health and Vitality

Health and vitality are not destinations but continual journeys. Embracing this notion involves acknowledging that well-being is a constant process of development, learning, and adaptability. By adopting a mentality that emphasizes tenacity and lifetime commitment, you may negotiate the ebbs and flows of your health journey with resilience and grace. Here's how to embrace the constant path of health and vitality.

1. Understanding the Journey

1.1. Lifelong Commitment

Ongoing Process:

- Continuous Learning: Health and vitality demand a dedication to continual learning. Stay updated about new research, trends, and practices that can boost your well-being.
- Evolving objectives: Understand that your health objectives will develop over time. As you mature, your requirements and priorities will change, prompting you to modify your approach.

1.2. Dynamic Nature

Adapt and Adjust:

- Flexibility: Embrace flexibility in your health path. Life events, changes in circumstances, and new problems will require you to alter your techniques and goals.
- Resilience: Cultivate resilience to face setbacks and challenges. Recognize that ups and downs are part of the process and that tenacity is vital.

2. Cultivating a Growth Mindset

2.1. Embracing Change

Positive Outlook:

- Growth-Oriented: Adopt a growth mentality that views problems as opportunities for progress. Believe in your potential to gain new talents and conquer challenges.
- Openness to Change: Be open to modifying your habits, routines, and techniques. Embrace new experiences and be open to experimenting with different ways to find what works best for you.

2.2. Learning from Experiences

Reflective Practice:

- Self-Reflection: Regularly reflect on your experiences, triumphs, and setbacks. Use these thoughts to acquire insights and make informed improvements.
- Input: Seek input from others, such as healthcare experts, trainers, or support groups. Use this feedback to boost your understanding and improve your practices.

3. Building Sustainable Habits

3.1. Consistency and Routine

Establishing Habits:

- Routine Development: Create daily and weekly routines that complement your health objectives. Consistent practices are the cornerstone of long-term well-being.
- Sustainable Practices: Focus on building sustainable practices that you can continue over the long run. Avoid excessive diets or fitness programs that are difficult to continue.

3.2. Incremental Progress

Small Steps:

- Gradual Changes: Implement changes gradually. Small, gradual actions are more doable and less daunting, leading to sustained improvement.
- Appreciate Milestones: Recognize and appreciate your progress along the road. Celebrating little accomplishments may enhance motivation and promote positive behavior.

4. Nurturing Holistic Well-being

4.1. Integrating Wellness Dimensions

Balanced Approach:

- Physical Health: Prioritize regular physical exercise, balanced nutrition, and appropriate rest to preserve physical vigor.

- Mental and Emotional Health: Practice mindfulness, stress management, and emotional resilience to support mental and emotional well-being.

- Social ties: Cultivate meaningful relationships and social ties to boost your sense of belonging and support.

4.2. Holistic Practices

Comprehensive Care:

- Mind-Body Connection: Recognize the connection of physical, mental, and emotional well-being. Adopt activities that foster all elements of your well-being, such as yoga, meditation, or holistic therapy.

- Preventive Care: Focus on preventative measures, such as frequent health tests, good lifestyle choices, and proactive self-care.

5. Staying Inspired and Motivated

5.1. Personal Inspiration

Finding Joy:

- Passion and Interests: Engage in activities and interests that offer you joy and contentment. Pursuing hobbies may increase your general well-being and keep you engaged.
- Positive Role Models: Look up to role models who exemplify health and energy. Their tales and experiences might inspire and drive you on your quest.

5.2. Community and Support

Collective Effort:

- Support Networks: Build a network of supporting friends, family, and communities who share your dedication to health. Their support and accountability might help you stay on track.
- Shared objectives: Participate in group activities, workshops, or challenges that correspond with your health objectives. Collective activities can provide a sense of solidarity and inspiration.

Embracing the continuing path of health and vitality includes knowing that well-being is a dynamic, lifelong process. By creating a growth mindset, building sustainable habits, nourishing overall well-being, and staying energized, you may traverse your health path with resilience and tenacity. Remember that every step, no matter how tiny, contributes to your total success. Celebrate your triumphs, learn from your experiences, and stay dedicated to your goal of a healthy, vibrant life.